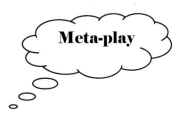

The Meta-play™

MANUAL:

Theory-based Interventions
For Young Children
With Autism

Cooper R. Woodard, PhD, BCBA

ISBN 978-1-4675-5141-0

Table of Contents

Introduction

In my first book, *The Meta-play Method: Application of the Dynamic Behavior Theory of Autism (DBTA)*, I spent a great deal of time explaining what we currently know about autism and how this knowledge led to the creation of DBTA. For example, it was essential for the reader to not only know the core symptoms of autism, but also the many unusual associated symptoms. Symptoms such as limited make-believe play and the reversal or absence of pronouns are typically not focused on, but give important clues if our goal is to create a working theory of what autism is and where it comes from. In my first book, I also discussed what is known about genes and environment and as expected, experts in the field are now suggesting that twin research over-estimated the role of genetics (Dawson, 2012). In other words, the role of genetics may not be as strong as we once thought, leaving us to focus (luckily) on something we can control more easily, the environment.

I also discussed what is currently known about effective treatment, and then quickly turned to early development and the "9-month revolution" in thinking. I did this not only for the obvious reason that autism by definition emerges prior to age 3, but also because the absence of behaviors that emerge around the first birthday are important in making a diagnosis of autism. For these reasons I, like many other researchers, have focused on this critical, yet somewhat mysterious and complex point in development that takes place just before the first birthday in typically developing children. We reviewed a number of theories to better understand the mechanism for the emergence of what we ended up terming the ability to "think about," meta-represent, or imagine, but the theories did not offer a full or satisfying explanation of this early period or how it related to the cause of autism.

I conceived of autism as the cascading effects of impairment in the early emergence of this ability, and suggested that <u>object-</u> versus <u>person-based</u> identification was at the core. I hypothesized that children with autism come predisposed to identify with objects, and as a result, do not internalize a model with "thinking about" abilities. Rather, they come to think in a more object-based manner. Without the human model, the abilities to think in a more sophisticated and abstract way do not develop. In addition to the object-human continuum, we suggested a continuum of <u>part</u> to <u>whole</u> thinking, and postulated four possible trajectories that loosely correlated with various presentations of the person with autism.

While there was no research directly available to support this new theory, there was research that indirectly supported it. For example, more and more research suggests that very young children with autism fail to orient to biological motion, such as dots representing a person walking (Klin et al., 2009). Instead, these children chose to look at non-social, physical attributes that were also present in the visual field. Simply put, children with autism preferred the physical, object world to the social, human world. With these ideas in mind, it follows then that to create autism (which of course we don't want to do), one might try to induce a culture-wide focus on objects to the detriment of human contact. This is a situation that I suggest has, in fact, taken place, and may be one contributing element to the rise in autism that has been observed in the past 20 years.

The final section of my first book delineated a set of activities that emerged from DBTA, and were termed these the "Meta-play Method." At best, these were rough sketches of interventions that we piloted with one participant, although we were encouraged when this participant lost his autism diagnosis after only 6 months of treatment. Since that time, we have been able to revise, expand, and refine these interventions, as well as organize them in progressive sequences for ease of understanding and implementation. We have also embedded these interventions in the larger, ongoing, environmental "good ideas" put forth by leaders in the field of early, effective treatment, with the goal of creating a "perfect storm" in the battle to defeat autism. The interventions of the Meta-play Method draw on the novel DBTA theory to augment current treatments that tend to "coax" or "wait for" the child with autism to behave in the desired manner; Meta-play Method interventions give the parent or practitioner something he or she can actually do, and needs to do on an ongoing basis.

Because research designed to test the efficacy of Meta-play Method activities or interventions is ongoing, I cannot yet state that Meta-play Method interventions are effective and empirically validated. But once our research is complete, it will be submitted for publication regardless of outcome. A recent article (Dawson et al., 2012) demonstrated the efficacy of the Denver Early Start Model in improving IQ scores and measures in related areas, but this model failed to affect core severity ratings of autism to a significant degree (Note that diagnoses however, were altered in the desired direction). While this is impressive, the central goal of research on the Meta-play Method is to reduce or eliminate the core symptoms that create autism; a goal that has been elusive to say the least.

The present book begins with a brief review of DBTA in the simplest and most general manner possible. (For readers interested in a more thorough description of the theoretical basis of DBTA or more information on the ideas noted above, please see my first book.) The goal of the review is to introduce readers to the theory, or remind readers of our first book of the theory's main concepts. Because the Meta-play Method incorporates the principles of applied behavior analysis (ABA) into the theoretical base, the second part of this book introduces the reader to behavioral procedures essential to implementation of the Meta-play Method. ABA procedures have been empirically shown to be effective in the field of autism, and are a key element of my method. Finally, the third section of this book expands upon the Meta-play Method interventions from book one, and begins with interventions that can be ongoing, in contrast to the progressive, sequential interventions that follow. These more structured interventions are discussed in detailed form, with six activities in each of two chapters. Finally, I have included some of the monitoring tools that we developed for our research, so that parents can monitor and evaluate their child's progress.

In summary, this book was written for parents of children with autism, and for practitioners working with young children on the autism spectrum. The interventions of the Meta-play Method described within are designed to foster the child with autism's ability to "think about" by refocusing the child with autism's attention from objects to people and from parts to wholes. The activities are designed to help create the thinking that supports desired behaviors, or the behaviors that may ignite more sophisticated thinking "realizations." The interventions draw from scientists and effective practitioners in the fields of applied behavior analysis, early development, psychoanalysis, and early treatment of autism spectrum disorders, with the goal of bringing all there is to bear on the unusual group of devastating symptoms known as autism.

A special thanks to some special people who have helped with this book and supported me in research efforts: Jin Chung for her continual moral, technological, and conceptual assistance, Leslie Weidenman for her excellent editing and proof-reading skills, my parents for listening and helping create materials, and Lisa Rego and June Groden for believing in this project.

Cooper Woodard

July, 2012

Part I: **The Basics of the Dynamic Behavior Theory of Autism (DBTA)**

Chapter 1:   The Origins of DBTA

Becoming acquainted with the core ideas of the Dynamic Behavior Theory of Autism (DBTA) is important for two reasons. First, you will implement the interventions more effectively if you understand <u>why</u> you are doing <u>what</u> you are doing. In a related vein, the effects of what we are proposing may be subtle and demonstrated in a variety of ways, so if you understand the "why," you will be better able to spot the subtle changes that we are trying to bring forth. Second, the interventions described in the final section of this book may need to be adapted or altered to fit your child's particular and unique needs, preferences, and interests. By understanding the "why," you will likely be better able to make changes which maintain the original, theory-based core ideas.

So, let's review the basics of DBTA. Autism has a small group of core symptoms such as impaired social engagement, impaired communication, and repetitive or restricted interests, as well many associated symptoms. These associated symptoms don't fit nicely into the core symptom group, and perpetually perplex the autism researcher (and most anyone else involved with persons with this disorder). For example, why is make-believe play often impaired or inhibited in the person with autism, and how does it fit into the core symptoms? Is it a social impairment? Communication impairment? Repetitive behavior? I would suggest that it is none of these. In another example, why is pronoun use often impaired? Why not verbs or nouns? What is it about pronouns in particular, and how can we conceive of autism in a way that accounts for this and other very unique symptoms?

So we know that autism is not composed of a simple and straight-forward group of symptoms. We also know very little about where autism comes from and how it develops, although this minimal knowledge is not from a lack of trying. On the contrary, extensive research exists on the roles of genes, environment, and even early

11

treatment. Genetic research has found some consistent patterns in a small subgroup of persons with autism, but the general consensus seems to be complex, combinations of genes, that may somehow give rise to autism "vulnerability." In other words, we have some promising leads, but there is no smoking gun. Environmentally, we have yet to locate any one element or "toxin" that is responsible for the emergence of autism. This also is not the result of a lack of trying; a host of possible toxins have been suggested, but none have stood up to rigorous research so as to be identified as a cause of autism.

And finally, as far as treatment is concerned, we know that to affect the fundamental symptoms of autism, intervention needs to be early and intensive. This is not particularly surprising for a disorder that by definition must be diagnosed by age 3, but what types of interventions have worked? Applied behavior analysis (ABA) has been shown to be very helpful in numerous studies, and interventions incorporating ABA procedures such as Pivotal Response Treatment (PRT) and the Early Start Denver Model (ESDM) have shown success. These treatment models employ intensive parent training with 1:1 therapies that are designed to address core or "pivotal" areas of autism. In addition, these treatments capitalize on teaching strategies that focus on maximizing positive social interactions, and both verbal and non-verbal communication. But what do we mean by "success"? In a recent article on ESDM efficacy, the IQ of children with autism improved after treatment, but scores of the severity of autism did not improve significantly (Dawson et al., 2010).

One of the strengths of the ESDM however, is its focus on all developmental domains, meaning that the approach and techniques are based on what we know about typical child development. Similarly, DBTA makes use of what we know about typical development. Also, much like PRT and ESDM, behavioral principles and parent training/implementation are essential features of the approach/application of DBTA. Specifically, there is a point in early child development so significant in terms of cognitive changes and development, that it has been termed the "9-month revolution" by developmental theorists and researchers. (For background references and information on this area, please see our first book.)This important step in development signals the emergence of the ability to "think about," "meta-represent," or simply and broadly, "imagine."

When considering these "internal" events, it is important to identify the actual behaviors that are emerging or changing that leads to such abstract hypotheses. Around the first birthday, this revolution in thinking is demonstrated by the child's ability to attend to the emotional expressions of others (often called social referencing), attend to people and objects in a joint manner with another person, use objects functionally, to share enjoyment with others, and even point or show items to another person. My theory suggests that essential to all of these behaviors is the ability to meta-represent, "think about," or imagine. I would suggest that later developing skill areas are likewise dependent on this ability. I use the term "imagination" to refer to this broad concept that is fully discussed in our first book. Specifically, the emergence of language, recall, pretend/symbolic play, and even the use of pronouns is suggested to be reliant on the emergence of earlier imaginative or thinking "about" abilities. But don't take my word for it. Many developmental theorists have discussed these changes in thinking; Piaget, Tomasello, Stern, Fonagy and others. The perspectives and ideas (and references) of these theorists are outlined in my first book for the interested reader.

An absence of the very behaviors that signal the 9-month revolution in thinking is significant in that children not demonstrating such skills typically get a diagnosis of autism. For this reason, we scoured the work of theorists listed above for mechanisms, to see if we could identify the manner by which this "revolution" comes about. While each suggested their own perspective on this area, it wasn't until the work of Peter Hobson was considered that other possibilities came into view. Peter Hobson (2002) suggested that infants came into the world "innately equipped" to "identify" with another person. By this, Hobson meant that infants took on another person's "stance" or "characteristics," and as a result were "lifted out" of dyadic (child and object or person) thinking into the world of triadic thinking (child, object, person, and thought about that other object or person); namely, imagination. Using what we know and don't know about autism, and expanding on this concept of identification, DBTA was created.

Chapter 2:   Identification, Object-relations, and DBTA
              in a Nutshell

Expanding upon Hobson's conceptualization of identification, I reviewed and integrated concepts from the psychoanalytic literature. Specifically, more than assuming a "characteristic" of another person, when I use the term "identification" I mean an actual psychological merger or unification with (typically) someone else or (less typically) something else. In the psychoanalytic school of "object relations," this someone or something else is called an "object." Further and according to psychoanalytic theory, when the infant identifies or merges psychologically with this "object," he or she mentally internalizes not only the object itself, but subsequently the relationship with that object. So this internalization first serves to become the "thinking template" by which other people and events in the outside world are viewed or perceived. In other words, by internalizing and merging with the other person, that person's manner of thinking becomes the child's manner of thinking; then the relationship with that person becomes a more central issue. Not surprisingly, people often engage in therapy (or self-reflection) only to find that they have been interacting with the world and others in it consistent with these early experiences. This is the "stuff" of the school of psychoanalytic thinking called "object-relations."

For our purposes, we are concerned with the initial, early process of primary identification, where the origins of the infant's subjective world emerge from this other-person-based unification. In simpler terms, the infant uses (temporarily) someone or something else to make sense of early psychological chaos, and create a way to organize the self, and learn to think. It follows then, that the 'object" selected is important indeed; much like the right prescription for your glasses determines how you will see the world, the object that is selected for internalization "lays the track" for the very foundations of thinking. Further, in object relations, the object selected typically progresses from a <u>part</u>-object to a more integrated <u>whole</u>-object state. In the case of primary identification, we could use this concept in a nearly literal sense: the perception of "parts" of the other person or thing in contrast to perception of a "whole" person or thing.

The core idea of DBTA is that autism is the result of impaired, thinking "about" or imagination abilities, due to early identification with a part, physical object instead of a whole person. This idea is a combination of developmental and psychoanalytic perspectives. The treatment application adds the third essential component, the behavioral perspective. By combining these orientations, we hope to not only create a theory that accounts for much of what we know about autism, but also make possible a focused intervention in the treatment of this disorder. As a special note, I know that psychoanalytic thinking and autism do not share a particularly positive past. For this reason, I will again point out what was clearly stated in my first book: I would suggest that the child comes into the world predisposed to identify with objects versus people. It is not any action or inaction on the part of the parent that causes autism. Typically, infants effortlessly identify with humans, yet for reasons unknown, the infant may not always "choose" such a trajectory.

<u>Part</u>- or <u>whole</u>-identification with an <u>object</u> or <u>person</u> is not suggested to be an all or nothing, black or white event. On the contrary, I am suggesting that this concept is best viewed as taking place on a continuum from part-object to whole-human. In my first book, four main demarcations of identification were suggested and are discussed in detail. In the present text, I will only note their existence for the purpose of communicating a special facet of DBTA: It is a continuum approach that allows for the many varied presentations seen in persons with autism. The demarcations are not however, random combinations of symptoms; they are progressive groups drawn from and consistent with DBTA. As such, they could and should be evaluated empirically. Because

DBTA is a new theory, it is essential that such research take place not only to evaluate these hypothesized demarcations, but also to add research-based information to what was presented in our 2012 book.

One final concept that was discussed in the first book is the relation of DBTA to the ever-increasing rate of autism. The same way we hope to apply our theory to produce interventions to decrease autism, we also can use the theory to speculate (and this is pure speculation) on what factors might increase the severity and/or prevalence of autism. With the main concepts of DBTA in mind, how might we hypothetically intervene or alter a culture so that this disorder was fostered (which of course we don't want to do, which is why this is a hypothetical question)? Based on DBTA, we would focus on increasing a culture-wide focus on and/or interaction with physical objects. Further, we might want to "pump up" the possible effect by adding a co-occurring decrease in person-to-person social contact. We might start by training adults in this fashion, and then move on to adolescents and children. The purpose of this would be to effectively increase object interest and decrease social/affective skills in tomorrow's parents. Better yet, if you made professional success in part dependent on higher object focus, the people who are naturally (and genetically) good at this would be more likely to engage with each other, and produce offspring with such a genetic predisposition.

I would suggest that this scenario is exactly what has happened in the past 50 to 75 years. People used to have no choice but to have social, person-to-person contact to live and progress. As time went on however, technology helped to "speed things up" by putting an end to the need for actual social interactions. Instead, we were given the telephone, television, and a curious object that has increasingly taken up more and more of our time, the computer. So, instead of walking into the next office and talking with someone face to face, I send an email or leave a voicemail. Instead of telling someone about my trip to

Boston and showing my pictures, I post them on my social networking site and type comments about them. I engage in texting instead of calling and talking to another person. Instead of going on a walk or enjoying dinner with someone, I sit with my face buried in my phone. (Surely you have seen this many times as I have.) What is common to all of these situations? Object focus is pursued at the cost of social, face-to-face, one-on-one interaction.

Based on DBTA, such a culture-wide phenomenon should create over time, an increased prevalence of autism. Further, there would be no "toxin" to be found, and genetics/studies would suggest a combination of complex genetic contributors to the problem: the link would only be in the genetic or biological sources that affect our desire to object-focus and/or our ability to engage socially at a very early age. I would suggest that there is a possibility that this is what is happening in our culture today, and it is a problem that will only increase if we maintain object focus to the detriment of social engagement. One way to test this theory would be to compare the prevalence of autism in a "developed" country to the prevalence of autism in an area untouched by technology. If someone could actually find an area untouched by technology, that in and of itself would be impressive.

Part II: **The Necessary Basics of Learning Theory and**
Applied Behavior Analysis (ABA) Principles

Chapter 3:   The ABC's of Behavior, Reinforcement,
              and Prompting

        Now that we have had a review of the origins of
DBTA as well as the core concepts of this theory, it is time
to add to what we have put forth regarding the
developmental and psychoanalytic perspectives. As stated
previously, the third "arm" or component of DBTA is
behavioral principles and technologies. This component is
necessary to translate DBTA into application. This chapter
and the next are devoted to cover the behavioral principles
that are necessary for successful implementation of the
interventions that compose the Meta-play Method. In
combination with chapters 1 and 2, the reader should be
well-prepared not only to understand why the Meta-play
Method activities are what they are, but also how might
add to or adapt these interventions to maximize any
potential effect.

        So let's start at the beginning and state that
applied behavior analysis (ABA) is a set of guiding
principles or ideas that are based on learning theory and
related research. For many decades, researchers in this
area have been studying **behaviors**, mainly because
behavior involves action and can be observed by others.
In contrast, internal states or events such as anxiety,
confusion, or thinking, can't be seen by another person.
These internal events are only knowable to the person
experiencing them. A behavioral psychologist won't say
that these don't exist, only that since they can't be
observed, they are hard to measure or verify. Behavioral
psychologists do note many behaviors that suggest
internal events, such as a furrowed brow indicating worry,
or holding one's arm indicating pain. Because we want
psychology to be a science, we need to be able to
measure and verify what we are studying, so behaviors
and only behaviors become our central data of interest. As
such, behaviors are certainly important and in need of
discussion and explanation, but remember our discussions

from chapters 1 and 2: our behavioral interventions will (as you will see in Section III) be specially selected and designed to affect thinking, focus, and identification.

Behavioral psychologists and learning theorists have carefully defined their concepts in very specific and technical language. For example, a distinction is made between behaviors that are voluntary and those that are involuntary. Much of what we will focus on consists of voluntary behaviors which are termed "**operant**" behaviors by learning theorists. (Involuntary behaviors are what are commonly called reflexes.) This class of voluntary behaviors is also known as "instrumental" behaviors, although you will quickly notice that neither term, "operant" or "instrumental," really tell you much about what this class of behaviors are about. In any event, operant behaviors are simply those that at some point, you <u>choose</u> to do. As a result of the voluntary behavior or action, usually something happens. For example, when you wave your hand at someone they will typically wave back, or when you flip a light switch, the light comes on. What this **consequence** is and how it affects that behavior you performed is the nuts and bolts of behavior analysis and learning theory.

Events that happen in your environment have an influence on the behaviors you choose to perform. Events that happen before a behavior are called antecedents, and if they are present often or always before the behavior you performed, we start thinking of that particular antecedent as a "trigger." "Trigger" is not a behavioral term, however we are interested in this consistent relationship between **antecedent (A)** and **behavior (B)**. The **consequence** of your behavior is luckily a word that begins with "C," so typically we behaviorists see the world in A-B-C relations or contingencies. Once we know the relationships between the antecedents (A's) and consequences (C's) for any given person's behavior (B), we can (and do) adjust the A's and the C's to change the B's that we are interested in, either to increase them or decrease them.

Sometimes a behavior is called a "response," which should not be confused with a consequence. When you hear the word "response," it means a behavioral response to an antecedent event. This is just one of those things that seems to be designed to confuse people.

So we have a behavior that is something someone chooses to do, and this behavior (B) often has things that happen before it, the antecedents or "A's", and things that happen after it, the consequences or "C's". The simplest place to begin examining relationships among A-B-C's is with the consequences or "C". It is easy to recognize that if you like the thing that happens after you perform a certain behavior, you will likely do it again. You are also likely to notice that if you perform a certain behavior and as a result, something you don't like to do (such as a chore like dusting) is taken off your plate, you will also likely do that behavior again. When the frequency of a behavior increases as a result of these types of consequences, we call them **positive reinforcers**, and the ones we didn't like that were taken away, **negative reinforcers**. Negative reinforcer is a term that can be very confusing and is often used incorrectly. When you see the word "negative," it seems like something bad, but in this situation it is a good thing. In the behavioral world "positive" simply means "applied," and "negative" means "removed." Any "reinforcer" always increases behavior, so a negative reinforcer indicates an increase in behavior because you removed something unpleasant. It's like another language, isn't it? The important point to remember though is that these terms are defined only by the effect that they have on the rate, frequency, duration, or intensity of the behavior of interest.

Here are some examples of reinforcement. I buy a winning lottery ticket at a certain convenience store after I see another "winner" on a TV ad. The antecedent is the TV ad, the behavior is going to the convenience store to buy lottery tickets and the consequence is winning money. Because I won money it is likely that I will go back to that same convenience store and buy more lottery tickets. Since my behavior of buying lottery tickets increased, the winning of money would be a positive reinforcer. If, on the other hand, I never went back to buy another ticket, although we always want to call winning money a positive reinforcer, in this case it would not be a positive reinforcer because the behavior did not increase. For an example of a negative reinforcer, I think about taking off a tight shoe. A tight shoe is uncomfortable, and when you take it off, your foot feels much better. As a result of that experience, whenever you have a tight shoe on, you are likely to take it off as soon as possible. Because an unpleasant state was removed by the behavior of removing the shoe and this behavior increased as a result, the relation meets the definition of negative reinforcement. Notice that with negative reinforcement something unpleasant or "aversive" must be occurring, which we don't like to do from an ethical standpoint. That's why we try to focus first on positive versus negative reinforcement.

Before we talk about how to deliver positive reinforcers so they work effectively, let's **operationally define** a behavior. What we mean by this is clearly identifying a behavior so everyone can agree on whether or not it occurred. This makes the behavior easier to count, and if you and I agree that it occurred, we will have good **inter-observer agreement** or **IOA**. In section III, one activity involves choosing the most human-like picture out of three cards. The group of three pictures is often called an **array**. What exactly is the behavior I want to happen? Do I want you to point to the right card? Touch it? Hand it to me? When we operationally define a behavior, we state exactly what we want to have happen. In this example, I will say that the behavior I want to take place is for you to hand me the most human-like card. When you place that card in my hand within 3 seconds of my giving you the instruction or **prompt**, we will agree that the desired behavior has taken place.

In terms of A-B-C's, an instructional prompt took place ("Pick one!") which is the antecedent, and you handed me the card within 3 seconds which is the behavior. Because I want you to do this again, I need to give you a positive reinforcer quickly, and I know you like pretzels so I give you one. In the next trial, you pick the correct one again, so now I know that pretzels are, in fact, a positive reinforcer for you. Notice I said that I had to give you the pretzel very quickly; why is that? Well, reinforcement works better if you give it right after the behavior that you want to increase occurs. So, however you choose to find your reinforcers, by using surveys or just observing, deliver them quickly! Also, it helps to change the reinforcers occasionally to keep things "fresh." Even if I love pretzels, too many can get boring which in behavioral terms is **satiation**. Finally, be sure to give reinforcement on a consistent basis, especially when you are trying to get a new behavior to catch on. This helps to really cement the behavior; then you can reinforce more intermittently to maintain the behavior.

On the other hand, if you want a certain behavior to decrease, the consequence would need to be a **punisher**. For most people, this term brings images of spanking and other aversive consequences, but remember that in behavior analysis, terms are defined only by the effect they have on rates, frequency, duration, or intensity of behaviors. The same is true for punishment, so if a behavior rate decreases as a result of a certain consequence, that consequence is a punisher. It doesn't matter if the consequence that (we presume) caused this behavior change is a pinch or a marshmallow; if the behavior decreases, it is a punisher. One final simple term before we go on to the next chapter is **discriminative stimulus** or "S^D." A discriminative stimulus is like a signal that indicates some behavior will be reinforced, such as picking up a ringing phone. Or, remember in the three-card array I mentioned that the instructional prompt in this example was "Pick one"? When the person picks the correct card in the presence of those words and only those words, this prompt is called the discriminative stimulus. The reason for this is that by performing the correct behavior when given this prompt and only this prompt, we are saying that he or she is then able to discriminate between this prompt and other similar prompts. By the way, this is an example of a "verbal prompt." Other types of prompts include (in order of increasing intrusiveness) "gestural" where the instructor might point to the array of cards or even the correct card, "partial physical" where the instructor lightly guides the learner to the correct behavior (or "response"), or "full physical" where the instructor gives full physical guidance so the correct behavior occurs. In the next chapter we will move on to another important set of behavioral concepts.

Chapter 4:   Functional Behavior Assessment, Shaping,
              Discrete Trial Training, and Teaching
              Strategies

The purpose of the previous chapter was to
introduce you to some of the more basic concepts of
applied behavior analysis, and this chapter builds on those
ideas. For example, we discussed how the selection of a
certain consequence may serve to decrease the rate of a
behavior, which by definition means it is a punisher.
Another way to decrease the rate of a behavior is to
withhold reinforcement. When someone has been getting
reinforcement for performing a certain behavior and then
the reinforcement stops, the behavior usually stops too. If
this happens, we say **extinction** has taken place. A
common example is a child tantrumming because in the
past, this behavior has succeeded in getting the child what
he or she wants. If the reinforcement is withheld and the
child doesn't get what he or she wants, after a short
increase, the rate of behavior should begin to decrease. If
this happens, we say the behavior is "extinguishing" or
"extinguished" ("Extincted" is not a word, by the way!).

Many of these concepts or ideas seem obvious;
they occur regularly in our human experience. But
identifying the obvious and creating a structured science
based on what seems so evident now is an impressive
feat. That's why the people who identified them (e.g.,
Skinner) are considered some of the greatest thinkers of all
time. Another thing you may have noticed is that if you can
figure out why someone is doing what they are doing,
selecting effective interventions becomes easier. It turns
out that behaviorists realized this a few decades ago, and
decided to call the process of figuring out the purpose of
behavior **functional behavior assessment** or FBA. There
are a number of ways to do an FBA (interviews, recording
behavior sequences, or setting up certain situations to see
if the behavior occurs), but the easiest way is to select the
behavior you are interested in, and write down what

happens immediately before and after. Typically this process will show you the purpose or "function" of a behavior, with the main functions being 1) the child doesn't feel well or has a medical problem, 2) escaping or avoiding something, 3) to get attention, 4) to get something tangible like a toy or food, or 5) just because the behavior feels good (or **automatic reinforcement**).

In our previous example of the child having tantrums to get things, we would say that the function of this behavior is to obtain something tangible. Now comes the tricky part. If you know the child is behaving in a certain way (i.e., having tantrums) for a certain purpose or function (to get tangibles), what should you do? The obvious answer (now that you know what "extinction" is) is to not give the child what he or she wants when the tantrums occur. That part is correct, but what else could you do? This is where **functionally-equivalent replacement behaviors** or **FERB**'s come in. A FERB gives the child an alternative to tantrums so he or she can learn how to get what is desired through more appropriate means. For example, the child could ask nicely or earn the money needed to get the desired item. When these preferred behavioral options are encouraged and reinforced, and the tantrum behavior is not effective any longer, the result can be a very effective behavioral "package." (Note however, that the extinction of the tantrum behavior is likely to be an ugly and difficult process!) Related closely to FERB's is functional communication training or FCT. In FCT, any form of communication (or any socially appropriate behavior) that meets the function of the original behavior is reinforced.

Usually when we want a behavior to take place, it doesn't just "pop on"; it has to be slowly shaped into existence. This process, not surprisingly, is called **shaping**. Let's say you want to teach someone to bounce a ball on the floor five times without stopping. If the person didn't understand verbal instructions, you would need to wait until he or she got <u>near</u> the ball. At that point you would reinforce! Then you would reinforce when the ball was touched. Then you would reinforce picking up and bouncing the ball, and so on until the person was bouncing the ball five consecutive times. You will notice that the person being shaped by you is successively getting closer and closer to the desired behavior, or approximating it. The teacher is said to be "shaping" the behavior, and the learner is making **successive approximations** to the desired behavior. Like shaping, if a person needs to learn a behavior with a lot of steps (such a setting the table), we would use a **chaining** procedure. This involves breaking the task down into steps, which is called a **task analysis**. Then we would teach each step either from the beginning using **forward chaining** where the learner performs the first step and then gets help with the rest, or from the end using **backward chaining** where the learner is helped right up until the last step which he or she performs independently.

When we are shaping a behavior or using chaining procedures, we need to decide what kind of prompts or assistance in learning we are going to provide. Often we start with full physical prompts, and then slowly reduce the amount of assistance. This "maximum to minimum" approach ensures that the correct behavior takes place early on in learning and that incorrect, non-desired behaviors don't creep in and spoil what we are trying to achieve. In teaching, we can also arrange the learning materials or other elements of the environment in a way that makes an incorrect response almost impossible. This process is called "errorless teaching," and it ensures our desired behavior gets on track right away. For example, if you want a child to pick a certain card, you might push that one slightly forward in addition to directing his or her hand to it. This makes an error almost impossible, and gets the learner going in the right direction almost immediately.

One of the other things that is a bit confusing about behavior analysis is that sometimes we are talking about increasing desired behaviors, and sometimes we are talking about decreasing non-desired behaviors. The reason for this is that some of our interventions are designed to do one thing (reinforcement increases behavior), and others are designed to do another thing (extinction and punishment decrease behavior). One concept that we have not discussed yet is kind of a combination of these ideas: **differential reinforcement of other behavior**, or **DRO**. When we use DRO's (sometimes the "O" stands for zero rather than "other" but it's the same idea), we are saying that we are reinforcing any behavior "other" than the non-desired behavior. If the non-desired behavior occurs, we don't' reinforce it, so technically speaking, it is being "extinguished." There are other forms of differential reinforcement such as a DRA (differential reinforcement of "alternative" behavior), but the idea in each of these is very much the same as the original. You are reinforcing the child when the undesired behavior does not occur.

In the next section of this book, we will use many of these principles and procedures to foster certain behaviors from your child. Additionally, there are some related procedures that we need to mention here in preparation. The first one is **Discrete Trial Training**, or **DTT**. In DTT, we use many of the procedures or concepts we have already discussed to optimize the learning of a certain behavior. In DTT, we start by reducing distractions in the environment, and making sure we have all of our materials ready (e.g., the three cards and a reinforcer if we are using DTT to have a child pick the most human-like card). We seat ourselves across from or next to the child (whichever you think will be less distracting), make sure he or she is paying attention, lay out the three cards, and present our instruction (or S^D): "Pick one!" This S^D is going to be paired initially with a physical prompt, where you help the learning with hand-over-hand guidance to put the correct card in your hand. Then you give a reinforcer, mix up the cards out of sight of the learner, and start again.

When you start this process, the learner usually can't help but do it correctly, because typically (but not always) you are physically guiding him or her. DTT sessions are usually 10 trials per session, so for the second set, you would "fade" the prompt. **Fading** is the process by which prompts are gradually removed, so the S^D can finally be the thing that elicits the desired behavior. In DTT, we have a planned method for fading prompts which was mentioned earlier: usually a full physical, to partial physical, to gestural, or something similar to that, depending on what you're trying to teach. (If you are trying to teach the pronunciation of a word for example, the prompts would look very different.) Once the learner gets 2 or 3 sessions at 90% correct or better with a certain prompt, we reduce the prompt to the next level until all that is left is the S^D. This takes a bit of practice, but you can get good at it. For more information on this and all the procedures I have mentioned, I recommend "Behavior Analysis for Lasting Change," by Mayer, Sulzer-Azaroff, & Wallace, 2012.

We have two more important ideas to review, and then we can move on to implementation of our interventions. First, **modeling** is showing someone how to do something by demonstrating it. This seems pretty straight-forward, and typically I would mention here the need for the model to be similar to the person we are expecting to imitate the behavior, perceived as competent by the observer, and some other qualities. But the reason we are reviewing these behavioral principles is because they are particularly relevant to the next section and DBTA. In our theory, you will recall that children with autism had a) little interest in people, and b) no concept of self. Without an early concept of "me" and "you," imitation of real or video-models is unlikely if not impossible. In fact, a lack of imitation is one of the central diagnostic symptoms for early identification of autism. So what do we do? Because of this unique situation, our video-modeling needs to be adapted, and in the Meta-play Method, it is. All video-modeling is done from the child's perspective;

that is, what the child should be seeing and doing. Because the child with more severe autism does not have the working cognitive capacity to see someone else do something and then say "Hey, I should do that," we modify the videos so that kind of thinking isn't necessary. This will become clearer in Section III.

Our final important concept in preparation for Section III is **generalization**. This term can be used in a number of different ways, but for our purposes, the term of generalization we are concerned with has to do with our S^D's. What I mean by this is technically called **stimulus generalization**, which is an expansion or broadening of the antecedent stimuli that indicate a certain behavioral response is likely to be reinforced. More simply stated, stimulus generalization is when you broaden the things or events that signal a certain behavior should take place. In our 3 card array example, in addition to "Pick one!" being an S^D, you might want to broaden this instruction cue to something like "Choose one!" or "Pick the right one!" These would all be examples of successful generalization if the child still performs the correct response. I've included this concept because in our next section, you will be given a set of activities that you may have to adapt, change, or use generalization for the intervention to be optimized. For example, my picking up a real phone is an obvious S^D for a child to pick up a real phone. But what should the child do when I pick up a toy phone or a banana, put it to my ear and say "Hello"? You guessed it; "generalize" and continue to pick up the real phone that is set before them.

So now we have covered much of what you need to know about ABA to effectively use the interventions in Section III. If you want more information, there are many good textbooks and websites that vary in terms of technicality and reader-friendliness. But they all cover, in one way or another, the ideas we have reviewed in these two chapters. All of these ideas can be expanded upon, so if it is more information you seek, you won't have to look far. But these are the basics and what you will need for our purposes. Just one final note: I purposefully left out a number of more intrusive behavioral interventions typically reserved for problem behavior treatment that does not respond to more benign measures. These include procedures such as response cost, over-correction, exclusionary time out, and others. Information on these are also available elsewhere, but are best implemented with someone who knows about behavior analysis and who can help you implement appropriate techniques correctly.

<u>**Part III:**</u> **The Meta-play Method Interventions**

Chapter 5:   Using What Works, and Adding On

This section of the book focuses on the actual interventions that compose the Meta-play Method. It contains detailed instructions on implementing the interventions based on what was learned from the pilot study, which was briefly discussed in the first book. The results of the pilot study revealed what worked and what did not, and pointed out way to improve tracking implementation and progress over time. Remember that all of the activities we have created so far are intended to do one or more of the following:

1) Foster cognitive movement on the object-to-person continuum as represented by increased interest in or engagement with people.
2) Foster cognitive movement on the part-to-whole continuum as represented by increased interest in whole objects and then whole people.
3) Increase the ability to imagine, from more basic concepts such as continued object existence (also known as object permanence) to more sophisticated concepts such as the thinking, intent, or emotions of others.
4) Increase engagement in or tolerance of activities that are out of the child's control, and under the unpredictable, human control of others (in contrast to the generally predictable control of objects).

Our challenge has been to create activities that a toddler will engage in, and that parents can do on a regular basis that meet these targets. But you will notice that the four items listed above do overlap to an extent, with the one, core feature being to shift a child's focus from physical objects in the environment to people. If there is one idea to hold onto, that's the one. As a reminder, our theory suggests that early identification with people creates the workspace for "thinking about" or imagination, the absence of which denote the symptoms of autism.

We have reviewed our theory and some basic behavioral principles. Our next step in developing interventions based on DBTA and utilizing these principles was to look at specific behaviors we could measure. These were briefly discussed in section one, but need to be clearly identified to be of use. The behaviors that fail to develop and suggest an early diagnosis of autism include:

1) joint attention (engaging with object and parent in a me-you-object manner)
2) deferred imitation (repeating an observed behavior at a later date)
3) pointing
4) social referencing (looking at the parent's face to get a "read" on the situation)
5) social initiations (prompting the parent for social interactions)
6) acting on the intent of others
7) functional object use (using an item for its intended purpose (i.e., fork))
8) imitation (child doing what you do)
9) social engagement and shared gaze toward something in the environment

If these behaviors are missing or minimal, what we learned in Section II tells us that we should be shaping approximations of these behaviors, and then reinforcing these approximations. For example, if you see the slightest imitation, or the child putting a phone to the ear, or rudimentary pointing, behavior analysis would tell us that we should reinforce the behavior to increase the rate at which it is being displayed.

Of course this makes sense, and by all means, if your child does these things, reinforce them! But here is where ABA alone may not be sufficient to address the core symptoms of autism. Without a theoretical perspective that addresses why these behaviors are not occurring, the parent may be waiting a long time for these behaviors to be displayed. In fact, they may never be displayed by the child, and the best trained parent may have wasted valuable time waiting to implement well-intended techniques. I conceive of these early diagnostic behaviors as outcomes, and ABA makes use of learning theory to understand the contingent relations among these outcome behaviors and the respective antecedents and consequences. The principles of ABA have a wide application and many effective treatment models have made good use of the principles. So will we. But my message here is that a behavioral approach that only targets outcome behaviors may be insufficient on its own to alter the core features of autism. Although I recognize that the Meta-play Method has yet to prove its efficacy, DBTA suggests a deeper, more foundational layer of thinking that we hope to target.

Some of the more well-known treatment models for young children include the Koegels' Pivotal Response Training (or Treatment) (PRT), or the Early Start Denver Model (ESDM) (Dawson et al., 2012). These models have research-based evidence that supports the benefits of each, which is to say that to a degree, each of these can be helpful. (By "helpful," I mean that certain types of gains (e.g., cognitive) are made, yet gains in the core symptoms of autism itself remain generally elusive.) The reason I mention this, is that these models share some common aspects that are completely congruent with those of the Meta-play Method. In a nutshell, these models tell us that for treatment to be effective, it should include:

1) A basic understanding of ABA principles and how to apply them effectively, including reinforcement of the identified desired behaviors listed above;
2) Active and comprehensive parent training so that treatment can be ongoing across all domains of a child's experience;
3) Novelty of experience to keep things interesting, based on the interests, cues, and choices demonstrated by the child;

4) A focus on interpersonal exchanges, "real-world" activities, and shared engagement, marked by positive affect;
5) Clear and structured opportunities for learning, with an emphasis on fostering both verbal and non-verbal communication;

Who could argue with these? Each point is reasonable, and the underlying behavioral foundation that extends into socialization and communication domains is evident.

As I noted earlier, the main elements of effective treatment models are completely complimentary to those of the Meta-play Method. First, as I stated previously, if your child displays any approximations of the desired behaviors the absence of which we have identified as early diagnostic indicators for autism, reinforce them quickly and consistently. We want these behaviors to increase, and so if you observe any version of them emerging, even the most basic and primitive forms of the behavior, do something you know the child will like. If he or she likes cookies, give the child a cookie; but remember, although you may like social praise, that doesn't mean your child will. It is easy to give, but may actually be aversive to the child; be sure the reinforcer you choose is actually a reinforcer. Next, you are your child's main therapist. You will need this book and a Meta-play therapist or resource of some kind for good training to occur. We want you to implement this model as much as possible, and across all domains of your child's life.

The third general concept we support that is consistent with other effective models is novelty of experience, and using the child's interests to guide interactions. Based on this idea, we attempted to design a wide array of many different Meta-play activities. Not only is there a wide variety of options (so you can change things up to keep it interesting), but you can adapt the ideas (now that you understand the theory) based on the interests of your child. We encourage this! We know that if toddlers are not interested in something, they won't do it, so don't fight that battle. Pick activities your child wants to do or watch what the child is doing, think of our activity list, and implement an adapted version.

Finally, the last two elements of effective models (positive interpersonal exchanges and structured learning opportunities) are less central to what the Meta-play Method has been designed to achieve. Of course improving and increasing interpersonal exchanges and shared activities is a desired outcome, but DBTA has a defined reason for why this is not taking place. DBTA suggests it is the preference for objects over people and parts over wholes that are impairing cognitive development. This is not to say that if your child engages with you, that you should not respond and reinforce. On the contrary, if you have social engagement, reinforce it! Perhaps with time, social engagement that is reinforced will increase the child's interest in people. However, I would add that there may be an underlying reason why interpersonal exchanges are not taking place, and without affecting this underlying layer of thinking, we may be treating symptoms and not the core problem.

In terms of interpersonal engagement and exchanges, my hope is that these skills will emerge as the child's interest shifts from objects to people, and his or her ability to imagine the thinking, intent, and emotions of others will come "on line." These are the things that make other people of interest in the first place; why would you interact more with something that was really no different than any other object? In your child's current state of cognition, I am suggesting that this is the case. The same general approach is true as we consider some of the final elements suggested in effective treatment models: clear and structured opportunities for learning with a focus on communication in any form. Everyone benefits from clear learning opportunities, and if your child is attempting to approximate words or use pictures to communicate, great! But what if he or she isn't? What if progress is so slow that you are concerned that your child won't gain enough communication skill to function well in the world? Again, think about DBTA. Many forms of communication are dependent on imagination, dual-thinking, or thinking-about abilities because in communication, one thing "stands for" another. Whether it is a word, a picture, or a hand signal, each of these is a symbol that represents a thing or person or event.

To be able to use symbols, your child needs to be able to have this duality-of-thinking cognitive ability. So, like interpersonal exchanges, we are going to work on fostering this foundational ability by shifting identification from objects to people, from parts to wholes, and in any way we can get imagination or "thinking-about" to occur. Our hope is that by shifting this focus, we bring the core ability of symbolization to come "on line," and communication becomes possible and likely.

In the next chapter, we will begin discussing the individual activities designed to foster this ability, but there are some additional general ideas or techniques we can add to what we have discussed here. These can be implemented at any time, and as much or as little as the parent-therapist deems appropriate. First, we would like you to imitate or mirror the child's actions and emotions intermittently, for short periods of time. This will be most effective if you have the child's attention first, so he or she can notice you are doing or feeling what the child is doing or feeling. The goal of this "reversed imitation" (reversed because usually we wait until the child imitates your behavior and then we respond) procedure is to provide opportunities for the idea to occur to your child that you, as another person, are "like" the child: you too think, feel, and have ideas and intent. This procedure may feel particularly uncomfortable to you at first, but keep at it, and if possible, have another person observing to see how precise you are.

So what might this look like? I am not talking about regular play with your child (although this is fine too; just not the reversed imitation procedure). Specifically, this procedure involves you doing exactly what your child is doing, moving as he or she moves, and producing identical facial features. Instead of providing the "almost-the-same" approximations of your child's behaviors and feelings (as parents typically do with a very young child), this activity involves doing exactly the same thing. You may feel as if you are mimicking the child, and to a degree you are. But our purpose here is not to make fun of the child, but rather foster the realization that there are special objects in the world called "people," and these "people" have some very unique and important qualities. So if your child is running, run alongside him or her at precisely the same pace; if he or she picks up a leaf with his or her right hand, you pick up the leaf with your right hand; if your child is having a tantrum, you (for a short period) can have exactly the same tantrum. And if your child looks at you and wonders what the heck you are doing, great! At least now you have your child's attention. Chances are, like many of the Meta-play activities, initially your child won't like what you are doing. That is ok; it only means you are creating situations that may be challenging new thinking. Like most or all of the Meta-play activities, try them for short periods and for as long as your child will tolerate them cooperatively.

In addition to "reverse imitation" or mirroring, another activity that can take place at any time is "problem creation." Perhaps I could call this "problem-solving," but you are going to create the problem in hopes that the child will solve it. An ability that is entirely dependent on imagination and also impaired in children with autism is problem-solving. I would suggest to you that the reason for this is that to solve a problem, one needs to imagine various possibilities; but without the ability to imagine, this of course will be tough for your child. So of course we want to go slow and only create obstacles that are challenging enough; not too hard, but not too easy either. Specifically, what we would like you to do is create simple problems that your child can solve and then move on to more challenging ones as your child is able. For example, for an item out of reach, place a step-stool in the child's proximity to allow them the opportunity to reach the object by standing on it. Or, tie a string to a desired object and wait for the child to pull the string to get the object. Or, place an object out of reach and a short stick within reach, allowing the opportunity for the child to use the stick to pull the object towards him or her.

The possibilities are really endless for this particular procedure and dependent only on the parent's creativity and the child's particular interests. If your child begins to tantrum when you create these situations, that's ok; learning is tough. Remember our discussion about prompts and shaping: help the child along with some physical assistance to train the desired problem-solving behavior, and then fade your assistance over time. As you become familiar with the more specific activities in the next two sections, you might want to combine this procedure with other activities. For example, if you are warm in your house, gain your child's attention and combine the gesture for hot (waving your hand near your face) with the word "hot." See if your child will try to push the buttons for the air-conditioning; if he or she doesn't, help him or her push the buttons and show positive affect and relief from the heat. This would be an especially good example to try if your child likes buttons and button-pushing. But if your child likes boxes, create an obstacle with the box by putting something good inside and closing it up. If your child likes blankets, tie one up so your child needs to untie it to play with it. Combine this with hiding the blanket, and you have combined "problem creation/solving" with an activity that will be described in the next section! Now you are becoming a real Meta-play therapist!

The third set of activities that can be ongoing and implemented whenever possible involves the specialized videos created by you or by your Meta-play therapist. These videos are based loosely on the idea of video-modeling, but with DBTA in mind, we need to eliminate the concept of a model. Because there is impairment in imagination, the child with autism cannot and will not imagine him or herself as the model in the video. So, your Meta-play videos will be specifically designed from the child's visual perspective. Additionally, they will be designed to shift attention from objects to people, from parts to wholes, and designed to address key behaviors in which we want your child to engage. Some of these videos will complement the activities in the next section and some will not. But as we combed through the various desired behaviors with DBTA in mind, certain ones were well-suited to our adapted version of video models. First, social initiations where the child spontaneously initiates an interaction with you (preferably for the sheer joy of doing something together) or requesting something of you (help, an object or "tangible," etc.), are a set of behaviors that are really more an outcome of improved imagination skills. However, because we know so little about how "thinking about" or imagination develops, fostering the core skill may be just as valuable as fostering a more outcome-oriented behavior.

In the video, we begin with interactions with preferred objects and show them from the visual perspective of the child. That means in viewing the video, you would see just the hands of a person playing with blocks, not the whole person. Let's say the hand we see is trying to create a tower unsuccessfully. So, the video moves to the hand of a nearby adult. We know the child is thinking that this "part" of the adult might do the trick and fix the tower, but remember we want "whole-person" engagement. So the video-view moves from the hand to the person's face, backs up, and "sees" the person as a whole. Then and only then does the child's hand in the video (remember, we never actually see the child) request help. Other versions of this video would move towards social requests or initiation for the sheer enjoyment of joint play. Or, it could be designed to show requests for "help" with the use of pictures or other communication devices recommended by your behavior analyst.

The next behaviors that we felt were well-suited to video modeling from the child's perspective were pointing, giving, and showing. These behaviors as a group reflect an already established interest in people, and presume that the child has some concept of the thinking of others. In other words, if I am pointing at something, I am imagining that you will perceive it; if I am giving you something or showing you something, then I might be able to conceive of you needing, wanting, or having some interest in that something. Again, these are outcome behaviors dependent on the very skill (imagination) we are trying to foster, but sometimes understanding or realization comes from doing. This is similar to experiences that perhaps you yourself have had in the past. Practicing outcome behaviors, such as completing algebra problems, can lead to "a-ha" moments; algebra as a whole can suddenly "make sense."

Videos that demonstrate pointing, giving, and showing, like the social initiation/requesting videos, need to be from the child's perspective, and shift from objects to people. So, in pointing, the view starts with a hand playing with preferred objects. Then initially, the view shifts to other objects that the child also prefers. Now back to the original objects, and again to the out-of-reach other objects. Next, the view shifts to the nearby parent (you), who looks at the video camera with attention, and a hand pointing at the out-of-reach objects comes into view. The parent gets the objects and brings them to the child. The next video would be much the same, but show pointing for the sheer joy of informing the parent about something of interest to the child; there would be no implied need or intent as in the previous video. Giving and showing would follow much the same process:

- Objects first, from the child's visual perspective

- Then these objects are given or shown to an adult and something good happens (such as the parent smiling or giving the child a reinforcer)
- Finally, any object is given or shown to the parent and the parent shows thanks and interest, but does not reinforce

At this more sophisticated level, the parent's response is the reinforcer now that people are interesting and valued.

Before we move on to the activities in our next chapter, two unique points need to be mentioned. First, there are three activities in the next two chapters that also work well from a video-modeling standpoint, these include 1) Peek-a-boo (an extension of Fostering Imagined Existence (FIE)), 2) Acting on Intent (AOI), and 3) Putting People Together (PPT). When reviewing these activities, keep our video-modeling-from-the-child's-perspective idea in mind, and create these additional videos if possible. For example, play peek-a-boo from the child's visual perspective, demonstrate someone who has a need or intent that the viewer assists with (but we never see the viewer), or put puzzles or Mr. Potato-Head (© 2012, Hasbro) together again from the child's visual perspective. Second, one particular behavior that is amenable to our version of video-modeling is response to name: In video format, show a hand playing with preferred objects. Then, have someone call the child's name, and have the video-view shift to the parent. The parent says "Hi!" and the video-view shifts back to the objects. This is repeated 2-3 times.

So in summary, we want to encourage reinforcement of desired behaviors, or approximations of those behaviors, the absence of which suggests autism. We want to have you, the parent, be well-trained so that you can implement everything we are discussing as much as possible and across all life domains. We want to vary activities to keep things fresh and of interest to the child, and be supportive of any attempts to engage socially or communicate. We also want you to periodically engage in reverse imitation, and "problem creation/solving" to the extent you feel these are appropriate and possible. We want you to be creative in the development of obstacles while being sensitive to the child's ability to succeed in solving these contrived challenges. That is, the obstacles should be challenging, but not too challenging. And, finally, we want you to prompt viewing of the videos especially created for your child by you or your Meta-play therapist. These videos are designed to show your child the specific things we want him or her to do in a way he or she can understand. After viewing these videos, the goal would be to generalize the behavior to real-world situations: prompt the desired behaviors of social initiation, giving, showing, etc., by setting up real-world situations when they can happen. And remember to reinforce!

Chapter 6:   Meta-play Activities #1-6

The main differences between the three procedures reviewed in the previous section (mirroring/reverse imitation, and child-perspective video-modeling) and those to follow, are specificity and sequence. The activities in this section and the next are specific, meaning that they do not require development of original situations; they also occur in sequence, meaning that they are organized in a certain pattern or set of levels that organize the presentation. For each activity, I will briefly discuss the purpose or idea behind the intervention, and how it relates to DBTA. I do this so that if you do choose to modify the intervention, you can maintain the core concept behind the activity. After discussing the purpose, I will outline the activity in detail. Many people ask me how many of these activities should be done in any given day. Because we continue to test the efficacy of the Meta-play Method, my answer to this question is that you should integrate these activities as often as you can into the ongoing play of your child. Some other general rules include:

1) Start where your child shows an interest or success. If your child is not interested in the activity, he or she will not likely take part for any length of time.

2) Repeat activities over and over. It may take many trials of any given activity for new thinking to emerge.

3) Move along slowly if needed, and make slight changes only (such as a color change) if you think that your child is struggling with one of the activities.

4) Talk as you engage with your child and introduce activities. Say what you are doing as you do it, and point out the important parts. For example, when you hide an item, say "I know it is here somewhere!

Where could it be?" When putting the bear together, say "Now where does this leg go?" Try to pinpoint what you are doing with language on a regular basis.

Note that after we discuss all 12 activities in this chapter and the next, our final chapter will show you how to monitor which activities you are implementing on a daily basis, and some ways you can monitor your child's progress.

Activity 1: Pairing Reality with Representation (PRR)

Purpose: Recall that in DBTA, one of our goals was to prompt any behavior representative of imagination, starting with the most basic and/or object-based and moving on to more abstract or human-based. One way we can achieve this is to focus on symbolization, where one thing "stands for" another thing. To be able to do this, one needs the duality of thinking previously discussed and in our first book, so we begin in this activity with object-based imitation, and slowly move on to the more abstract. By doing this in sequence and slowly fading prompts, we hope to foster imagination/symbolization/thinking duality abilities in your child.

Activity Sequence/Instructions:
Level 1: At the most basic level, we want to pair any object-play that your child is engaging in with an identical object. So, if your child is playing with a real phone, the parent should play with an identical phone. If the child is playing with a real cup or using a real cup, the parent should do the same with an identical cup. If the child is playing with a certain toy, the parent plays with the same toy. The parent can engage in similar movements as the child, but the goal here is not the same as mirroring: you can simply play with an identical object in a similar way as the child, in as close proximity as possible. At this stage,

we want to catch the child's attention, and have him or her see that you both are doing similar things: this is the most basic introduction to duality. And these situations don't need to be limited to phones, cups, or toys. You can use any natural situation or context to match the object use of your child: using eating utensils or brushing teeth before bedtime are opportunities for level 1 PRR.

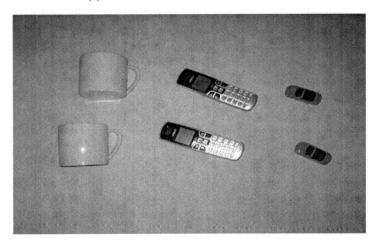

Level 2: At level 2 of PRR, we want to take one small step away from identical objects, and also add some people-based activities to the mix. If your child is playing with a real phone for example, you would introduce the use of a similar, play phone and engage in the same play or procedures as when you both used a real phone. You may need to physically guide or prompt this play to

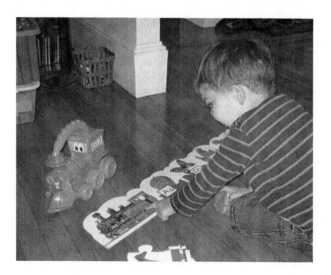

begin with by putting the real phone in your child's hand as you hold the toy phone, and then fade this prompt as possible. Try engaging in a phone "conversation," or just say "Hello!" and "Goodbye!", picking up and setting down the phone and toy phone. In our other examples, we want to replace your cup with a similar or toy cup, and your toy with a similar but different toy (a different size or color race car for example). The idea here is to prompt in the child's mind that one thing can be "like" or "stand for" another thing, laying the foundation for what we call imagination.

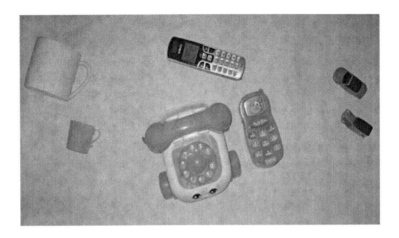

In addition to substituting "like" for "real" or identical in level 2 PRR, we want to introduce more people-based pairings to move the child towards people and away from objects. In addition to the activities noted above that involve objects, begin by engaging in parallel activities with your child such as running, or swinging on swings, or cooking with play cookware. When your child does these

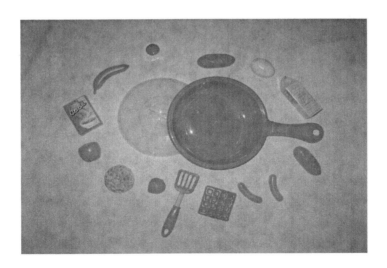

things you do them too, again trying to prompt the idea that you are "like" your child in many ways, and that there are two of you. Don't worry if your child stops engaging in the activity when you start; you are challenging your child to think in a different way by having him or her recognize the role of people and how one thing can be paired with or stand for another. These are ideas that your child would probably just as well prefer to avoid. Because of this, escape from these learning situations is to be expected. If this is the case, perhaps you could introduce your involvement by playing a bit further away from your child, or by engaging in the activity for an amount of time your child will tolerate. Keep trying and shape approximations toward the desired form of the behavior; and don't take refusals or escape behavior personally! Learning is hard work.

Level 3: Level 3 PRR takes any "like" item or activity, and pairs something much more abstract to the real item. For example, we take the toy phone one step further and substitute an abstract object for the toy phone. You might use a block or a banana as your "phone," when your child is using the real or toy phone. Do the same with other play situations, such as the cup/toy cup or toy/similar toy: if your child is driving a toy race-car, you would do the same with the block-as-race-car. Make the same sounds and movements, and prompt interactive play with your child as he or she will tolerate. At this point you may be able to reverse roles and have the child use the block-as-race-car (for example). If this does not happen naturally or spontaneously, physically prompt the use of the block while you use the real or toy version of the object you are playing with.

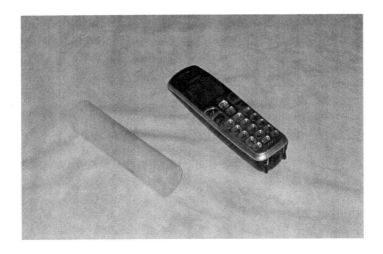

Level 3 PRR also adds an abstract version of people: dolls. When you are swinging on the swings with your child for example, have a human-like doll join you and your child in this activity. When engaged in object play, have the doll now be your substitute; the other "person" playing race-car with your child. Note that this is a particularly difficult concept for children on the autism spectrum to grasp and it is likely that they won't like this substitute doll at all. So, introduce it slowly and gently and keep trying to integrate the doll in small doses. At this point, I hope you are beginning to understand how DBTA combines with behavioral principles, not to treat the symptoms of autism but rather to treat the hypothesized core issue: impaired imagination, duality of thinking, symbolization, or "thinking about." As you have seen in this first example, we sequentially introduce the idea that an object can be represented by something else, as well as move from objects to people. We may need to physically prompt the desired behaviors and then fade these prompts as your child makes successive approximations to the desired behaviors, but that is to be expected: building the ability to "think about" is tough work! And as we discussed earlier and in my first book, it is likely

that your child simply came into the world with a desire to focus on objects and avoid this process in general. It is no one's fault and nothing you did or didn't do, but you can help your child to move in a different cognitive direction.

Activity 2: Fostering Imagined Existence (FIE)

Purpose: Knowing that an object continues to exist even though we can't see it is called object permanence. When you go to get something in your basement or garage, or when you search through your kitchen cabinets for an item, you are using and relying on this cognitive ability. Interestingly, searching for items is not typically something that people with autism do; once it is gone, it is gone. The exception to this is when someone with autism learns by repetition that when they open the cupboard, food is there, or when someone is farther along on the object-person continuum discussed in book one. In both these situations, it may appear that "searching" is intact and taking place on some level. But true searching that involves where an item "could" be requires imagination via hypothesizing (or "thinking about," or imagining) possible locations, and this is impaired. As a result, a person with autism will typically not continue to look in new and different possible locations.

This activity breaks down object permanence into 3 steps, and like activity #1 (PRR), then shifts from objects to people. The purpose or goal of this activity is to foster the ability to meta-represent objects, and then make this move from objects to people. In activity #1 our focus was on symbol representation, and in this activity we switch to fostering the imagination of objects and people not observed in the immediate environment. Our ultimate outcome goal is for your child to want to play games like hide-and-seek, or peek-a-boo.

Activity Sequence/Instructions:

Level 1: The simplest version of knowing that something continues to exist even though we are unable to see it would be to almost be able to see the object clearly. For this reason, we begin this sequence of activities with being able to almost see a desired object, and then training the behavior of removing the obstacle to obtaining that object. This is done with a set of three increasingly shaded boxes, but the initial goal is to train the child to lift the clear box and get what is underneath it. The sequence begins with the non-shaded box, and then moves on to increasingly shaded versions of the same box: Be sure to gain the child's attention with a desired object of some sort, be it a cookie or a toy. We used a toy car that after you shook it said something fun and then drove a short distance. Such an item promotes the idea of objects beginning the shift to people, in that objects typically don't talk or move spontaneously. This particular car had eyes and a mouth as well (so we preferred it to an edible for example), complementing another activity we will discuss soon.

Once you have the child's attention and hopefully some indication that he or she wants the item, place it under the non-shaded box and prompt the child to get the item by moving the box. If he or she doesn't do it spontaneously, use the most to least prompting sequence we discussed and physically assist the child to get the item. Practice this lessening the need for prompt assistance until the child can perform this behavior on his or her own. Then, move on to

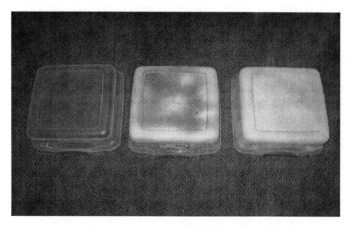

Box Sequence: Clear, partially shaded, and fully shaded

the partially shaded box, and move through the same sequence, gaining the child's attention and then reinforcing more and more independent attempts to get the item. The final stage of level 1 FIE involves the child learning to get the item under the fully-shaded box. At this stage the child is truly obtaining something that he or she is unable to see, pressing for the cognitive realization (or imagination) that objects continue to exist even though they are not visually present. This behavior can be generalized to many other situations and should be. Here are a few examples: When you are sitting at the dinner table, put a fork under the placemat with your child watching and prompt him or her to retrieve it. When you are getting your child dressed, hide his or her hat under the bed and see if the child will go to get it. If your child is playing with a toy, quickly put a blanket or towel over the toy and then assist to the extent necessary for the child to find it. When the child does find a hidden item, show surprise and make this an exciting game that the child will want to engage in time and time again.

Level 2: Once your child has mastered the fully-shaded box, move on to having the child see the object be hidden somewhere in the room. With the particular toy car noted above, we had the car "drive" under a blanket near the child, modeled getting the car ourselves, and then reinforced the successive approximations of the child performing this behavior. Then, as you might expect, we introduced people into the activity. We not only hid the car under the blanket, but had another person (a sibling in our pilot research) hide with the car. So in level 2 FIE, we challenge the child to expand his or her object permanence thinking to various locations beyond the boxes, and also add people to the objects. The goal here is not only increasing sophistication in thinking, but also shifting interest and attention from things to people. When both the person and the object are found (this may take some assistance from a third party), it is a big and exciting surprise that we want the child to enjoy. If possible, begin a sequence where the person and the object are given the opportunity to hide while the child counts with another person. This creates the routine for the next level of this activity set.

Level 3: When your child has the idea that you are hiding with the object in various locations and the process of finding you and the object is fun and exciting, we are ready to do away with the object and make this a solely person-based game. When level 2 behaviors are firmly in place, try having the child count with another person while you hide somewhere in the same room; don't make the challenge too difficult or your child might lose interest and go on to

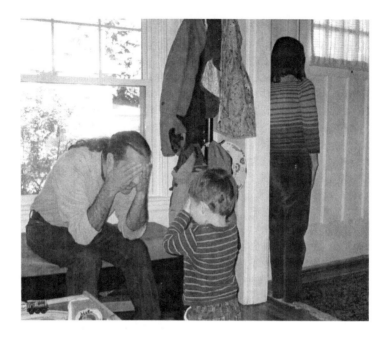

something else entirely. You may even want to allow the child to peek initially or leave a leg or arm visible, ensuring that he or she sees what is happening and finds you. Once you are in place, have the other person counting with your child help your child find you and experience with you the excitement that comes from this game. Note that for your child to engage in this game, he or she needs to "think about" where you might be. He or she needs to meta-represent or imagine objects at first, and then your existence. Your child needs to imagine the various places that you might be hiding, and because you have added yourself into the mix slowly and gently, will take an interest in people. Our hope is that this interest in people will grow, and at some point, it will occur to your child that you have thinking of your own; that's how you are coming up with these novel hiding places! This is a very human and very sophisticated version of imagination: knowing that you have thinking of your own!

Activity #3: Practice Unpredictable/Other-Controlled Play (PUP)

Purpose: In describing the ideas of DBTA , I talked not only about the object-to-person and part-to-whole continuum, but also what it might hypothetically mean to "be" or think like an object, and "be" or think like a person. Part of being or thinking like an object involves consistency: objects typically do the same thing over and over and are unlikely to engage in novel behaviors. When they do, we are pretty amazed and start thinking that there is something special or "human-like" about this object. One of the hypotheses about DBTA is that it is for this reason that children with autism enjoy engaging with objects instead of people, and will engage with objects in very repetitive or ritualized ways, doing the same thing over and over. Activity #3, PUP, targets this aspect of the developing mind and thinking preferences of the young child with autism, by exposing him or her to increasingly unpredictable toys and then shifting the focus to the experience of human volition or unpredictability in a tolerable way.

Activity Sequence/Instructions:
Level 1: As we noted above, most objects or toys do the same thing over and over, and this is preferred by children with autism. If there is something to spin or press or turn in a predictable way, that child will do it. If someone were to try to change the activity or remove the item, a problem behavior is likely to result. But there are toys that are less predictable than others, and there are ways that we could remove the child's control over those toys. For example, a ball usually rolls in the direction that someone pushes it. However, have you ever played with a ball that has a weight in it that is off center? This causes the ball to move in all sorts of unpredictable directions that we are unable to foresee. The same can be said of toys that are a bit more sophisticated, such as remote control cars or toys that can be programmed to do different things at different times. Having your child

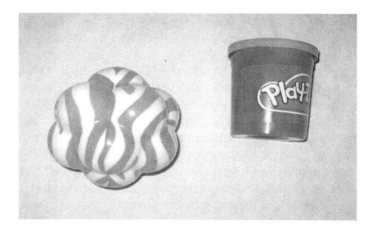

engage with these types of toys removes the possibility of repetitive play, and suggests that this toy may have a "mind of its own." This is a situation consistent with the concepts of DBTA and the goals of the Meta-play Model: prompting the possibility of imagination through situations.

Level 2: Now we want to introduce people and begin to decrease the role and importance of objects. The ultimate outcome of the PUP sequence of activities is the joy and enjoyment associated with the thinking abilities of others (as you will see in level 3). However in level 2, we would like you to pick up and move your child unexpectedly, in very short bursts that he or she will tolerate, or at least not have the time or opportunity to object to. You may want to begin with predictable movement, and then move on to less predictable and more surprising. So when your child is sitting in one seat, quickly and unexpectedly move him or her to another; when he or she is playing with a toy, quickly and unexpectedly turn him or her around to face the wrong way; as he or she is walking, scoop him or her up and move to a different spot. Similarly, you can "surprise" your child by popping out of places where he or she might not expect you. This should be done in as playful a manner as your child will tolerate, as we don't want to induce a fearful response.

Level 3: In the final phase of this sequence of activities, the parent moves on to swinging or "flying" the child in all different kinds of fun and unexpected directions. Be sure to physically support your child in a safe way, holding the torso fully and securely. Initially this will need to be done for very short periods, as the child with autism will undoubtedly not automatically enjoy the process. But the idea is that <u>you</u> are making the decisions on

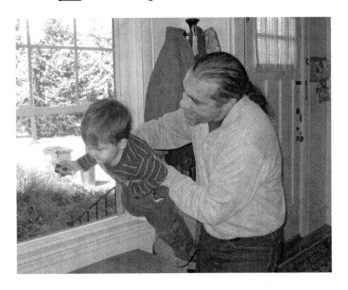

where you and the child are going, again creating the situation where the child is more likely to realize that you have thinking of your own: this would be something that would need to be imagined potentially, and therefore may be helpful to your child. The goal is to make the experience fun, and have the child imagine your thinking: You are the one thinking about what is going to happen next, and this situation sets the stage for such a realization. You might even say something like, "Hmmm...Where should we go next?" Or, see if your child can begin giving the instructions as to where to go and how fast or slow.

Similarly, you can create other situations where you become in control of the child's movement in a fun way. For example, you can place the child's feet on your feet, hold the child's hands and "walk" the child in all sorts of

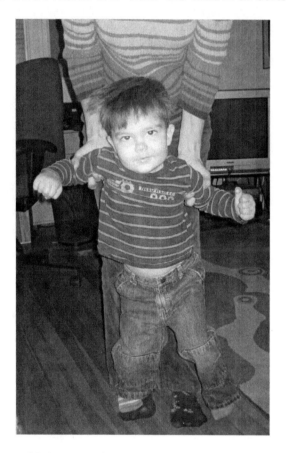

directions. Make sounds or move in unusual ways that increase the fun level of this activity. If your child likes to swim, when you are in the pool together, lift him or her up in the air at unexpected times, or count down to this interaction and "blast off!" The more unexpected the better, to the extent that your child will tolerate this type of interaction. And there is an added plus to this activity: Your child may begin to do what other children do to better predict future events: They will look at your face to try to get some idea of what is going to happen next.

Activity #4:   Restricting to Animal/People Play (RAP)

Purpose: One of the most basic ideas of DBTA is to shift focus from objects to people, even though children with autism really prefer to play with objects. You have probably noticed by now that the dolls and human-like objects in your household don't get equal playtime as objects that do the same thing over and over! For this reason, we want to create situations where we almost force engagement with objects that are "becoming" more and more human. We do this by organizing the sequence you see below, and then only making those objects available for periods of time (to the exclusion of anything else). You can model appropriate play during these times, and when interaction with a desired object takes place, remember to reinforce!

Activity Sequence/Instructions:
Level 1: At this initial level, we will allow some of the standard toys in the play area that your child has shown an interest in. Pick a few of the favorite toys, even if those toys have nothing to do with people. Then introduce some toys that have selected human features, but are still physical objects, such as cars with eyes, trains with faces, robot-like toys, or anything that combines object and human in any form. Slowly remove or fade out the favored object toys until just these human-ish toys are left, and

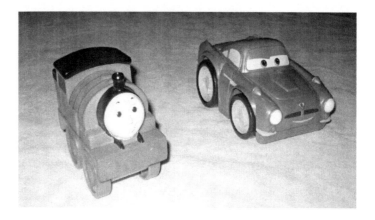

encourage play with these toys. Watch how your child plays with these toys; does he or she look at the faces at all? Does he or she enjoy making the ones that talk when you shake them or press a button, speak? Does he or she move or use the toy in any human-like way, like making it walk or "talk" to another toy? Model these types of behaviors for your child, or if possible, encourage cooperative play using the human features of the toy in your play.

Level 2: Once your child is accustomed to restricted play situations with the types of toys listed above, add more human-like toys. These could be dolls, or even stuffed animals with animal or human features. If your child will play with one of the toys listed above but resists these new toys, use them yourself and show how one of the dolls can ride the train, or how one of the animals can do what the doll is doing. The idea is to slowly introduce (and make appealing) people in contrast to physical objects, and challenge the child to (similar to the more advanced stages of the PRR activity) realize

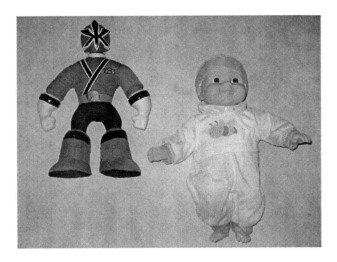

how a doll can be a symbol for a person. If possible,
introduce animal or human puppets here. Note, however,
that this initially may be unpleasant for children with
autism. This is because (we believe) that you are
introducing many elements that are contrary to their
preferred manner of thinking: people, representations of
people, and behavior that is not under the control of the
child. In our research, puppets were not initially cared for,
so you may want to introduce these slowly and stick to the
dolls if the puppets pose a sustained problem.

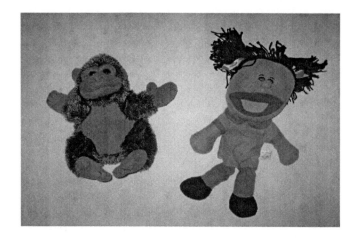

Level 3: The third level of activity #4 further reduces the human-like toys and restricts play to stuffed animals or human dolls. Again, if the child will engage cooperatively with puppets, then include those as well. But if not, reinforce any approximation of play with these toys. Try to insert yourself into this play situation with your child, and have him or her play with one doll as you play with another. Try to foster the two toys doing something together; start with

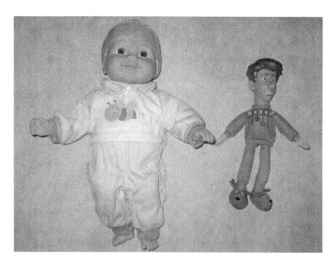

something simple at first, and then move on to something more complex. For example, the dolls may want to shake hands to start, and then move on to a cooperative activity like a tea party. This, however, is pretty advanced cognitively (representations of people engaging in pretend play), so you should be happy with your child simply tolerating exposure to these types of toys to the exclusion of the toys that he or she preferred. Remember to follow your child's lead and interests in this situation, and see what he or she will do.

Activity #5: Reinforced Putting People Together (PPT)

Purpose: Another basic idea of DBTA is to pay less attention to the parts of things, and instead start to see that parts put together make wholes. You may have noticed your child focusing intently on details or parts of toys to the exclusion of the whole. For example, he or she might play endlessly with the propeller of a plane, and never actually see that the propellor is attached to a much more interesting object that does much more interesting things. Or you might have noticed your child taking your hand and moving it somewhere to do something, as if the rest of you does not even exist. We want your child to see that your hand is part of a whole YOU, and that you are an interesting and special thing in the child's world that functions in a unique way. Note that for the activities below, introduce each item as a whole and take it apart in view of your child. That way, he or she will know what the item should look like at the finish of the activity.

Activity Sequence/Instructions:
Level 1: At this initial level, we make use of your child's likely interest in having certain items in his or her environment arranged or put together in a certain way. We will start with puzzles of objects in pieces or any physical, non-human object that you can find that needs to be put together. It doesn't have to be a puzzle; the couch needs

to be put together in a certain way, doesn't it? Certain household items are put together. A car that comes

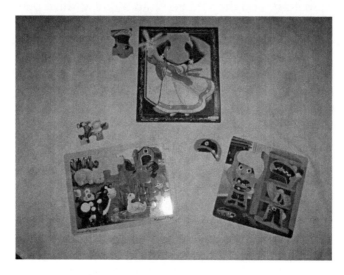

apart needs to be put together in a certain way too. This is not to be confused with "ordering" objects in the child's environment, such as putting books on a shelf in a tall to short pattern. Instead, we want activities with objects where the parts make a whole when assembled. A combination of toy-based items and real world items (like the couch example) are ideal.

Level 2: Next, we want to introduce the putting together of animal or human-like dolls or similar part-object and part-human toys. Below is an example of a bear in pieces which had small pieces of Velcro attached to the places where the arms and legs attached to the body. Initially

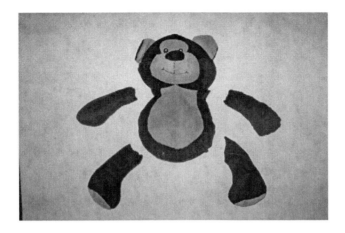

your child may put the bear together in an almost compulsive way, paying little attention to the whole bear that he or she is creating. That's ok! Remember that sometimes we have to engage in the behaviors before we realize the understanding of what we are doing. Or, you may have to reinforce one arm being put on, and then the next, building up to assembly of the whole object.

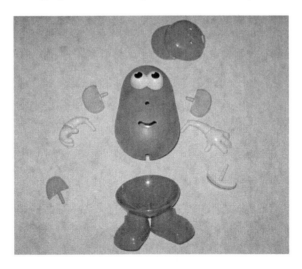

Another good example of this is a Mr. Potato-head (© 2012, Hasbro) toy because it is part human and part object, and challenges the child to put the essential parts of the body on the plastic potato. Or, try pop-up toys (see example below) that are in pieces when you press the button on the bottom, and then pop together when you let go. Whatever the child is interested in, follow his or her lead.

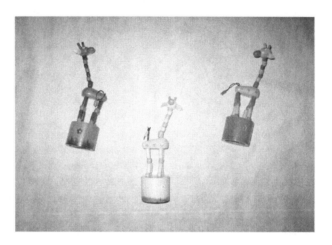

If you can find it, another good activity similar to these that we have discussed is the putting together of a doll with the physical likeness of the child (see example below). Remove the legs and arms of the doll, model putting the doll together as you did with the bear, and when your child puts it together, you can say, "Look! It's (insert child's name)!" While it may not happen the first time, this activity group not only challenges your child to put the world together, but draws his or her attention to people representations (dolls), and introduces the very cognitively challenging concept of "me." Whether you are working on the bear, Mr. Potato-head (© 2012, Hasbro), or dolls, look for any indication that the child understands what the whole is; he or she may suddenly try to animate the bear or doll, and make it walk for example. If this happens, be sure to reinforce it with excitement and positive comments! Your child is showing the primitive foundations of imagining and pretending.

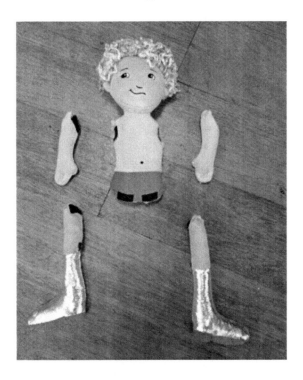

Level 3: When the child clearly can take part in these activities and is consistently putting together toys, animals, and dolls, introduce a puzzle picture of the child. Take a picture of the child or others in the family,

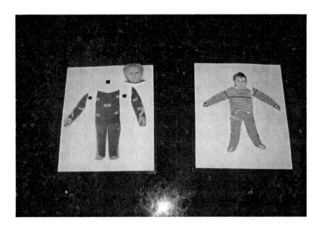

laminate it if you can, and then cut the arms, legs, and head off. Using Velcro, have the child put them back together as he or she would a puzzle. Challenge the child to "think about" this whole person: Ask him or her, "Who is this?" How can there be both me and a picture of me? This sequence of activities challenges the child to understand the importance of "wholes," not remain in a "part-based" world. It also challenges the child to understand that there are symbols or representations of the self and others. Wow!

Activity #6: Incidental Entertainment Training (IET)

Purpose: The idea in this set of activities is to use a form of media that some children are interested in to further the ideas of DBTA. Some children with autism watch TV and others do not, but if your child does, we want him or her to watch certain shows or videos. The reason for this is that many cartoons and animated features have entertaining examples of objects taking on human qualities; if this is a medium that has your child's attention, we want to make use of it. Specifically, we want to expose the child to any movie or show that ignites movement along the object-to-human continuum.

Activity Sequence/Instructions:
Level 1: Have the child start by watching videos where the objects are very people-like, or those where the objects are gaining approximations of human traits. Luckily, we have many good examples of these such as Thomas the Tank Engine (© 2012, Gullane), which seems to be a favorite of many children with autism. We are not sure why that is, but you will notice that the facial expressions of the trains are simple to understand, fairly stationary, and don't change quickly or suddenly. Additional examples of videos that we would place in level 1 include the human-like animals in Disney's "Bambi" or "The Lion King," or the very human cars (to the exclusion of any people at all in the

show) in Pixar's "Cars." In each of these, we have objects taking on human traits, thus beginning the desired shift from object to person in incidental situations where you might not be available to work with your child.

Level 2: In the second level of IET, we want to introduce people alongside the objects that have human-like traits. As in level 1, we are fortunate to have many good examples of these such as Disney's "Beauty and the Beast." In this particular story, we have people who, because of a spell, have become objects, yet they retain many of their human traits. That is what makes the show entertaining. But unlike "Cars," there are also people in this particular show, moving your child one more step towards becoming interested in people and less interested in objects. Other good examples of this include Pixar's "Toy Story" where toys come to life and are intermittently involved with people, and the Pixar movie "Wall-E®." In "Wall-E®," a robot has very human features indeed, and people are introduced later in the video.

Level 3: Our final suggestions for incidental entertainment that involves video viewing consistent with DBTA, consists of mainly people-based shows, with occasional objects that become people. Disney's "Alladin" is a good example of this, in that the main part of the video has people, and then animals are added with human-traits. Later, there is an object that comes to life with remarkably human features: the magic carpet. Not only do we have in this example a wonderful set of the process we are interested in, but the magic carpet displays many subtle and complex mannerisms that will be challenging for your child to interpret and understand.

These are the first six activities of the Meta-play Method, to be used as much as possible, depending on your time and availability and your child's interests. The idea of our purpose and how we made use of the concepts of DBTA in creating the Meta-play Method should be evident now. We want you to have that understanding, because you will need to keep the concepts that support the interventions described above active in your mind; they may need to be adapted by you to further our goals and purposes.   Next, we will turn to the other six activities that complete the entire Meta-play Method set as it is currently designed. The next six, similar to those described above are divided into levels so you have an understanding of the sequence. And, they are designed to foster imagination in the broadest sense of the word, re-focus interest away from objects and towards people, and encourage your child to put the parts together and see the "whole."

Chapter 7:   Meta-play Activities #7-12

Like the previous set of six activities, the next six are each designed in a progressive sequence of three levels. This organization helps those implementing the activities to better understand the idea behind each activity, as well as get an idea of what types of behaviors are ultimately the ones we want to see. You will notice that the final two activities are rather abstract and make use of pictures rather than three-dimensional objects. Your child might enjoy these types of stimuli or not; give them a try and see what happens. Typically, activities #11 and #12 are implemented last, but follow your child's lead and engage in the activities in which he or she shows an interest.

Activity #7: Parallel Puppet Play (PPP)

Purpose: Puppets and dolls are the ideal representation of a whole human being (or animal, depending on the puppet), and can engage in unpredictable, human-like play when a parent is "working" the puppet. A puppet behaves in a manner consistent with the thinking of the puppeteer, and in our pilot research, this combination of human and unpredictable features made the puppets particularly unappealing to our participant. But the goal is not only for the child to conceive of the puppet as a representation of the parents, but also to have the "thinking" of the puppet be imagined by the child. Because the child with autism is not likely to enjoy such stimuli or situations, we are going to begin with less aversive object puppets (created especially for the Meta-play Method), and fade in the features of a person so the child will be able to tolerate what typically developing children crave: the apparently unique and unpredictable thinking of a representation of another whole human being.

Activity Sequence/Instructions:

Level 1: In the initial level of this activity, you will be using puppets that have been specifically designed for the Meta-play Method, and might initially seem a bit curious to you. These are "object puppets" that have no human features, but rather are representative of a common object: a ball. The ball puppet will be the first puppet introduced to your

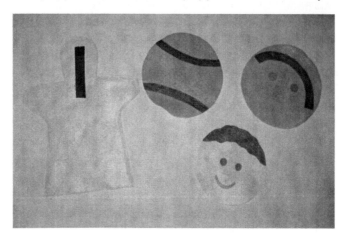

child, and because it is the first in a series, we don't want the ball puppet to display too much activity or "speak." We just want it to be present while your child is playing, and perhaps move closer and farther away from the child and his or her interactions with other toys. If your child attends to the puppet, try making the puppet engage in some simple manner with the child and the toy, but only approach the child as he or she will cooperatively tolerate. You may want to practice having the puppet engage in joint attention with the child and his or her toy, by not only being present, but "looking" back and forth between the toy and the child.

Level 2: In the second level of PPP, we will introduce more aspects of a person, and slowly fade these in to ongoing play activities. The puppet that has been designed for this activity set has a second "face" that can be attached to the main body of the puppet. You will notice that this second "face" has mostly aspects of the original ball, but also has the beginnings of a human set of eyes. Once your child is able to tolerate the ball puppet without any problems, switch to this half ball, half person face and engage in the same type of play activities as before. It will make more sense now to try joint attention activities, because your puppet now has "eyes." But try to refrain from going too quickly and adding speech to your puppet. We want to save that for the next level. Also at this second level of PPP, try introducing a small hand-puppet that the child might use, especially if he or she does not care for the larger puppets. The small hand puppet pictured below may help to introduce the idea that the child can create his or her own puppet representations, as well as create the "thinking" of this puppet.

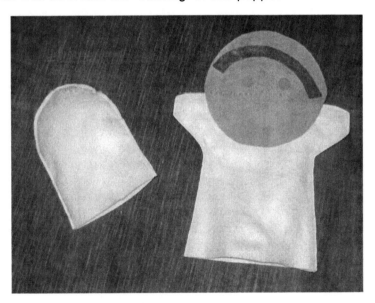

In addition to the second level face for your Meta-play Method puppet, you may want to try introducing animal puppets and see if your child will tolerate these. If your child has a favorite animal, like a cow or a chicken,

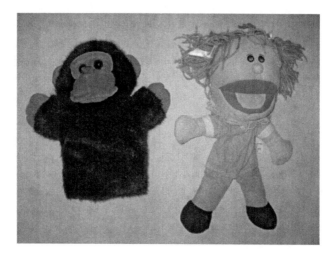

you may want to find a puppet along these lines and introduce it in play with your child. Remember that the goal is to introduce in an acceptable way the representations of people or animals that puppets are, and the unique and unpredictable thinking that they display through their behavior. Your child will need to cognitively make sense of this and imagine the thinking of the puppet, so this is a challenge that directly impacts the core ideas of DBTA.

Level 3: In level 3 of this activity, the puppets shift to completely human representations, and can begin to "speak" to the child. You can move to this level as soon as your child tolerates the puppets in level 2 which might have happened quickly or slowly. If it has not happened at all and you have been trying this for an extended period (one month or longer), you may want to try this third level anyway, and just have the human puppet engage from a distance. If the child is able to tolerate the level 3 human puppets, have the puppets speak and engage in active joint attention play with you and your child. Feel free to have the puppet "talk" to you and you respond, and then have the puppet "talk" to your child or otherwise engage with him or her in a playful and fun manner. If you are able to successfully get to level 3 and you are also pursuing the other activities in this section, you will notice that they can begin to overlap. For example, you could have the puppet need something or want to do something, and see if the child will meet that need or intent. These are the core ideas of #9 below.

Activity #8: What's in the Box? (WIB)

Purpose: If someone came up to you with a box with a hole in it and asked you to place your hand in the box, chances are you would not take part in this activity. Why? Because you can imagine all of the various things that could be in this box and the many things that could happen to your hand as a result of putting it in the box. This situation makes the WIB activity the perfect challenge for a toddler with autism. The purpose of this activity is to have the child with autism need to imagine in order to receive reinforcement, and then shift from more common physical objects to more human representations of objects.

Activity Sequence/Instructions:
Level 1: In level 1 of this activity, we want to simply acquaint your child with the WIB box; you can expect this not to go so well if our pilot research was representative of other children with autism. Get a medium-sized, cardboard box, about 1.5 feet square. Cut a hole big enough on one side for the child's arm, and another hole big enough on the other side for you to place items in the box. Begin by placing items the child wants in the box while the child is watching, and having him or her get the item through the hole on the opposite side of the box. You will need to reach through the big hole initially, and let the child see the item in the smaller hole. Remember that we need to shape towards the desired behavior and this is the first step. Don't worry if the child looks in the hole initially; we actually want that to happen because it means that he or she is

getting the idea that something continues to exist even though he or she can't see it. That means that the child is imagining.

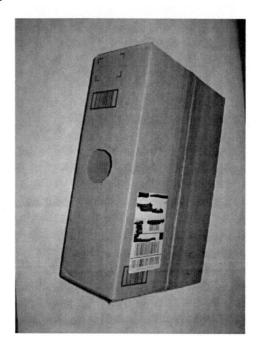

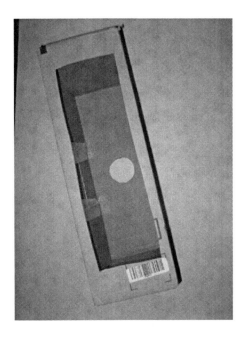

Level 2: The outcome of level 1 is the child reaching through the small hole to get items that he or she wants. Once this behavior is reliably taking place, put that same desired item in the box along with another non-desired item. The child will need to select their item from the set of two items, the one he or she wants and the distracter item. He or she may initially try to look in the smaller hole as before, and to start off with, that is fine. But as

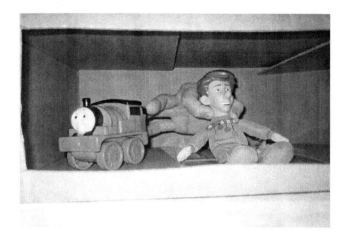

the child becomes accustomed to the activity, try to not let the child look in the hole or cover up the larger hole with a blanket or your body so it is dark inside the box.
Remember that this may initially be frustrating for the child, so you only want to make the activity as challenging as he or she will tolerate. You can always go back and show the desired item through the smaller hole if you think the child is losing interest or becoming overly frustrated.

Level 3: If your child is able to enage in level 2 cooperatively (and perhaps even comes to see the activity as fun), have the child choose his or her item from a choice of three. Make a big deal out of the child

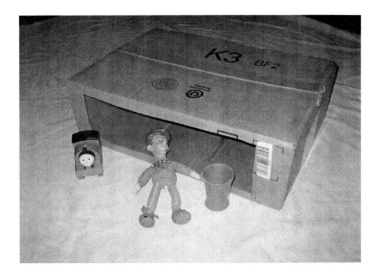

choosing the desired item in this situation! It is a big deal, because the child is actively imagining what he or she is handling inside the box. As this becomes more and more interactive and game-like, alter the game a bit and have the child move to choosing the more human object (such as a small doll) to get a reinforcer.

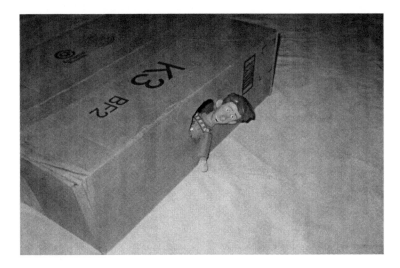

Activity #9: Acting on Other's Intent (AOI)

Purpose: As we mentioned above, an advanced goal is to get to higher levels of these activities which typically involves imagining the thinking of other people. The AOI activity does this by fostering the child's awareness and understanding of the thinking, intent, and/or needs of others. When you see someone reach for something for example, but it is just beyond that person's reach, you can imagine the intent of the person. If you so choose, you can get the item for that person and (hopefully) get reinforced for your kindness, but all of this behavior is dependent on your ability to imagine the intent of another person. We have suggested that the inability to do these types of things is at the core of impaired empathy that other practitioners have observed in persons with autism.

Activity Sequence/Instructions:
Level 1: Because this concept probably is foreign to your child, it is likely that prompting will be needed starting with full physical assistance. Start by creating a situation where you obviously need something or intend to do or get something. For example, if you are in the kitchen with your child, place a spoon or similar item out of your reach. Make it very obvious that you need the item and are reaching for it. Take your child's hand and have him or

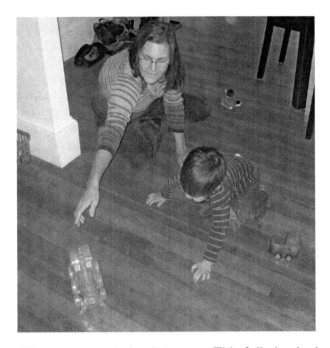

her get the spoon and give it to you. This full physical prompt is considered the most intensive prompt type. In response, be surprised and happy and give your child a reinforcer for engaging in this behavior. Remember to give your child the reinforcer quickly and consistently, especially when you are starting out.

Level 2: In the second level of this activity, fade away the full physical prompt and try to just use a partial physical prompt. Try this with the same situations that you practiced in level one. As your child becomes more likely to perform the behavior of giving you the desired item, fade your prompting more and more, but remember to give the reinforcer at the end of the desired behavior sequence.

Level 3: In level 3, you would again demonstrate the need or intent of the exact same situations, but don't give any physical prompts to your child. If your child is successfully engaging in the activity, you may want to try to generalize to other similar situations, such as reaching for a different item or in a different place. You can also begin to blend activities by having your puppets "need" things. You could even demonstrate the desired behavior by getting the desired item for your puppet while your child watches. Remember too that our ongoing, child-perspective video-modeling uses the AOI idea, so taken collectively, your child will have many teaching strategies that are focused on having him or her engage in behaviors that are representative of the thinking of others.

Activity #10: Object-to-Person Video-Modeling (OPV)

Purpose: We mentioned child-perspective video-modeling in chapter 5, which included initiating social interactions, requesting, pointing/giving/showing, and responding to name. In OPV which is, a 3-level sequenced activity, our only goal is to move attention from objects to people. It is what we considered to be one of the purest representations of DBTA, re-focusing interest from objects to people and using behavioral concepts such as reinforcement to increase the frequency of this trend.

Activity Sequence/Instructions:
Level 1: In the first video, we want to show interaction with objects from the child's perspective as was our practice in chapter 5. That means that the video actually shows hands interacting with preferred objects, and only hands, no fully human models. Then, only for a moment, the video moves to the face of the parent, and then back to the object. This can be in response to the parent calling the child's name as mentioned in chapter 5 or not. But the goal of this first step is to introduce the idea of a shift from objects to people.

Level 2: In level 2, we would incorporate the parent into joint play with a preferred object. Again the video would be taken from the perspective of the child; this would not be a video of the child and parent engaged with each other. Rather, there would be hands playing with objects, and then a view of the parent coming over and beginning playing with the objects. The child's view would shift between the objects and the parents face, and then to the parent playing cooperatively with the child and the toys.

Level 3: The third level of this activity would begin with examination of the face of the parent, demonstrating the primary interest that the child should have in the parent. Remember that this is from the child's view or perspective, so to begin with, this is a video of the parent's face saying something like, "Hi! Do you want to do something? I want to play with the cars!" Following this, the video would show joint play as in level 2. An advanced version of level 3 would include the parent saying, "Hey (child's name)! Do you want to see what you look like to me? " At that point the parent would, for the first time, take the camera and show the child in the video.

Activity #11: Most Human Card Game (MHC)

Purpose: Some of our participants in the pilot study were interested in cards and pictures, and some wanted nothing to do with them. So you might want to try this activity early on and then again a bit later if your child does not show an interest in these types of materials. In MHC, we have pictures of objects that fade to people, that have been specifically designed based on DBTA for the Meta-play Method. The purpose of this activity is to reinforce the child for identifying and choosing the most human version, creating this concept for the child to generalize to the real-world. Below are the car and cup sequences of pictures that are used in this activity set. They are arranged in least-to-most human order:

Car Series

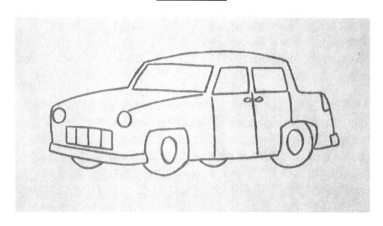

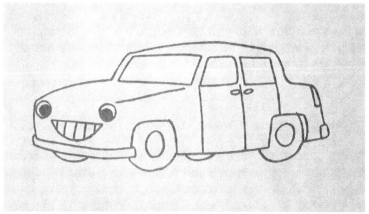

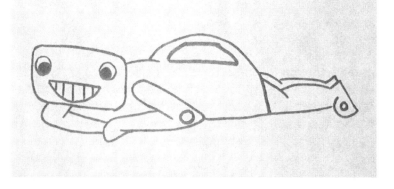

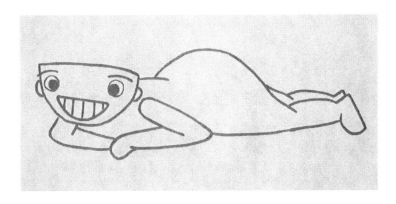

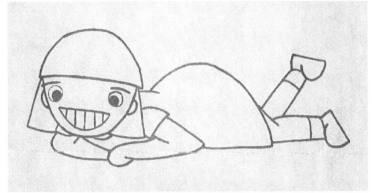

Original artwork by Hee Jin Chung

Cup Series

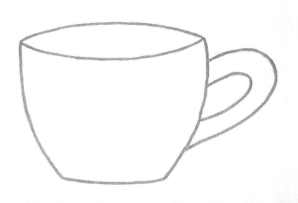

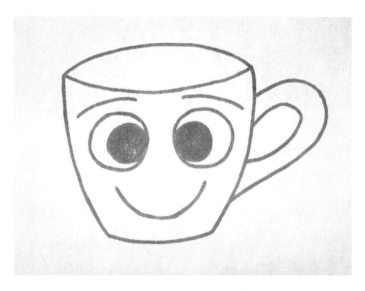

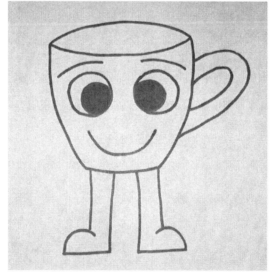

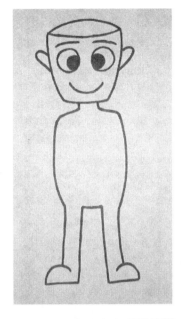

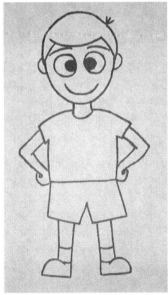

Original artwork by Hee Jin Chung

Activity Sequence/Instructions:
Level 1: We want to begin this activity as simply as possible, and the use what we know about DTT to maximize learning. So, we begin with a picture of an object, either the actual cup or car shown in the Meta-play Method MHC card series, and two distracter cards. The goal is to have the child reliably pick the card out of this array of three. Remember to reinforce

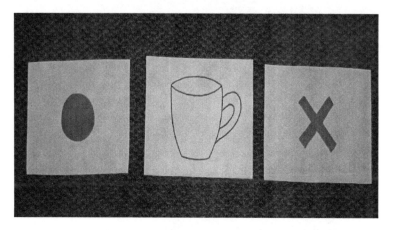

correct selections, and if the child selects the distracter card, shuffle the cards and use physical guidance to have the child select the correct card. Then try it again, perhaps moving the correct card a bit closer to your child to ensure the correct response.

Level 2: Once your child is selecting the object card from the array of three noted above, replace one of the distracter cards with the next most human card. Use the DTT teaching strategy to teach your child that the correct selection is the slightly more human card. Continue to introduce increasingly human cards with the original object card and a distracter card until the child can reliably select the most human card from any combination presented.

Level 3: In level 3 of MHC, the distracter cards are eliminated, and your child's challenge is to select the most human card out of an array of three cards, none of which are a distracter. One example of this presentation is displayed below:

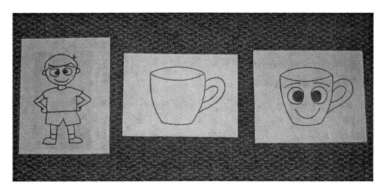

Activity #12:   Pairing Reality with Representation – 2
                (PRR-2)

Purpose: In PRR activity #1 presented earlier, our goal was to prompt any behavior representative of imagination, starting with the most basic and/or object-based and moving on to more abstract or human-based. We did this by pairing increasingly symbolic objects with real ones in natural contexts, and reinforcing the selection or use of the more symbolic object. PRR-2 is a DTT version of this idea, where we challenge the child to select the most symbolic version of the real object from an array of three.

Activity Sequence/Instructions:
Level 1: Place the actual object on a table, a phone for example, along with an identical picture of the object and 2 distracter pictures (a star and circle for example) in front of your child. From this array of 3 cards, instruct your child to "Match!" and start by physically helping him or her to pick the card that matches the object. If your child is interested in the cards and understands that the picture matches the actual object, he or she should, with practice, select the correct card. If your child chooses the correct card, reinforce! If not, then try it again and use physical prompts to ensure that the child selects the correct card. As your

child selects the correct card more and more reliably, fade your physical prompt to a partial physical prompt, and then don't prompt at all.

Level 2: Next, instead of the real phone picture, substitute the toy phone picture and repeat the process in level 1. The child now should see in front of him or her,

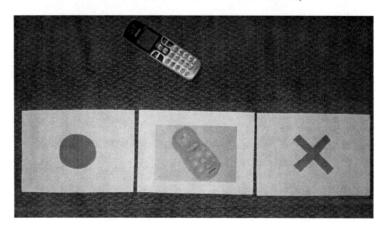

the real phone, a picture of a toy phone, and two distracter cards. The goal is to have the child select the toy phone picture from the array of three. Use the same instruction ("Match!"), remember to reinforce correct selections, and go back to full physical prompts if the child makes a mistake.

Level 3: Level 3 introduces an even more abstract version or representation of the phone in picture form, and continues with the DTT learning format. Instead of the toy phone picture, substitute a picture of an object that the child could use as a pretend phone such as a phone-length block or banana. Use the same procedure outlined in levels 1 and 2, with the ultimate goal being the child selecting this very abstract version of the phone in the presence of the real phone. This DTT version of PRR should complement the real world version described in activity #1.

Chapter 8:   Objectively Monitoring Progress

One of the biggest challenges when implementing interventions of any kind is to accurately assess whether or not the participant is making progress. This is especially difficult with young children with autism, for two reasons. First, young children continue to develop in varied ways, and sometimes what looks like a delay one day may not be a concern only a short time later. Different children develop at different rates, and children are famous for "catching up" spontaneously. The second reason has to do with the diagnostic indicators of autism itself. These are not clear cut, present or not present skills that can be simply assessed. Rather, the best (often called "gold-standard") tests for autism present various situations for the young child and then areas such as social engagement or joint attention are rated for frequency and quality. As there is an element of subjectivity in rating these behaviors, it can be hard to get high inter-observer agreement on the test score. Evaluators often need to work with each other to ensure the rating that he or she is giving is fair and accurate.

As a parent, you are not likely to have access to repeated, formal testing for your child, but if you do, typically these tests are only administered at one year intervals or slightly more frequently. That leaves a lot of time between such assessments. For this reason, we created a rating scale for our research that was adapted from a clinical scale used in previous studies. In addition, we outlined the various levels of the activities described in the previous chapters, and also created a tracking form so parents could monitor the type and rate of activity that they were implementing. Finally, we created a fidelity check which is a form that another person completes while watching you implement the activity. The purpose of this is to ensure that you are implementing the activity correctly and the way the activity was originally designed. With these forms, you have a quick reference to determine where you are in the progression of any given activity, and how much and how well that activity is being practiced with your child. **All of the forms below are available on single pages at our website: www.meta-play.com.**

The first form lists the activities in a table format. It allows you to see the various activities at each level of the DBTA intervention:

Intervention	Level 1: Object	Level 2: Object + Person	Level 3: Whole Person
PRR-1	Phone with phone Cup with cup Toy with toy	Phone with toy phone Cup with toy cup Toy with similar toy Parallel activities without objects (being on the swings with your child etc.)	Phone with block Cup with block Toy with block Doll uses an object or engages in a parallel activity
FIE	Three box activity	Hiding in a room and/with person	Hide a person in the room
PUP	Non-predictable toys (remote-controlled cars) Modeling clay	Move child unexpectedly/ surprised	"Flying child"; guided walking

RAP	Objects in play area that are human-like (like robots, half-human half object toy)	Add human objects (e.g., dolls)	Human toys and people only
PPT	Puzzles of object or people	3D: Mr. Potato Head(© 2012, Hasbro)/doll/bear	Puzzles of pictures of family or self
IET	Cars; Thomas the Train ©; Bambi; Lion King	Beauty and the Beast; Toy Story; Wall-E®	Aladdin
PPP	Object puppet	Object-person puppet; Bear/ Gorilla	People puppet
WIB (reinforcement)	Shaping any preferred object	Choice from 2 (I person + 1 object) no looking Person/object choice with no looking	Pick person from 3 items
Acting on others' intent (AOI)	Demonstrate need or intent (physical prompt)	Demonstrate need or intent (verbal/gestural prompt)	Demon-strate need or intent (No prompt)

OPV	Look from object to face Response to name	Joint attention with objects and people	Facial examination of parent engaging in activity
Most Human Card Game (MHC)	Real object card and two of the simplest distracters	Combinations of different levels of object-to-human cards in groups of 3	Most human card out of the array of 3, with neither of the simplest distracters
PRR-2	Real phone with picture of real phone and two distracters	Real phone with picture of toy phone with two distracters	Real phone with picture of block or banana with two distracters

Because there are so many activities and each has a set of levels, it can get confusing to remember where you are in each! But remember that the implementation of any of these activities is potentially helpful, so you really can't make a mistake.

The next form allows you to keep track of what you and other people in your household are doing in terms of implementation of these activities. Remember that more is better, and you may want to skip from activity to activity to keep things fresh and interesting for your toddler. The following form is designed to be used weekly, and we suggest that you post it somewhere where everyone in your home who is involved in treatment can give input. You will notice that on this form, we have the 12 activities that compose the sequenced activities of the Meta-play Method, and then follow this with the group of activities that can be ongoing and implemented/presented as often as you see fit. Implementation also depends on your child's cooperation level, interest, and general mood.

Weekly Log for Parents

Child's Name:_____   **Dates:**_____

Activity \ Day (Date)	S	M	T	W	T	F	S
PRR-1 (Pairing real objects with toy objects or block)							
FIE (Hiding objects to hide-and-seek)							
PUP (Unpredictable play like flying)							
RAP (Play with only human-like or animal toys)							
PPT (Puzzles of objects: Mr. Potato head (© 2012, Hasbro) etc.)							
IET (Movies with human-like characters)							
PPP (Object and people puppets in joint play)							
WIB (What's in the Box?)							

AOI (Parent demonstrates need and fades prompt)							
OPV (Video shifting focus from object to human)							
MHC (Pick the most human card)							
PRR-2 (Match real objects to abstract pictures)							
Mirroring child's emotion							
Problem creation							
Video modeling ☐ Social initiation ☐ Point/give/show ☐ Peek-a-boo ☐ AOI ☐ PPT							
SUM							

In addition to knowing the rate (frequency within a certain amount of time) with which you are implementing the activities, you will want to be sure you are doing them correctly. For this reason, it is helpful to work as a team if there are two parents in the home, or someone else in the home who is familiar with the activity set. Perhaps once or twice per month, have that other person complete the following form and give you feedback on how well and how accurately you are implementing the activity. We called this a fidelity check form, because we are interested in the quality and accuracy of implementation:

Fidelity Check

1. **General Impression** (e.g., progress, problem, etc.).

2. **Activities**

Level/ Check Activity	Lev 1	Lev 2	Lev 3	√	X
1) PRR-1 (Pairing real objects with toy objects or block)					
Comments.					
2) FIE (Hiding objects to hide-and-seek)					
Comments.					
3) PUP (Unpredictable play like flying)					
Comments.					
4) RAP (Play with only human-like or animal toys)					
Comments.					
5) PPT (Puzzles of objects: Mr. Potato head (© 2012, Hasbro) etc.)					
Comments.					
6) IET (Movies with human-like characters)					

Comments.				
7) PPP (Object and people puppets in joint play)				
Comments.				
8) WIB (What's in the Box?)				
Comments.				
9) AOI (Parent demonstrates need and fades prompt)				
Comments.				
10) OPV (Videos to shift attention objects to people)				
Comments:				
11) MHC (Pick the most human card out of the 3)				
Comments:				
12) PRR-2 (Match real objects to abstract pictures)				
Comments:				

Not only will this form help you be sure you are doing the activities correctly, but it also helps to keep track of what level you are working on. The "check" mark indicates the activity was done correctly, and the "X" indicates it was not and needed to be corrected. By completing the form regularly, you will be better able to track your child's progress. There is also an area for comments, so if you run into a problem or question, you can mark that down and access a Meta-play therapist with your concern.

The final form is one that we suggest you complete each month. It is a clinical impression scale that was modified significantly from an adapted autism version of the original (NIMH, 1985; Sandler et al., 1999) to address our areas of interest. It would be ideal if you could have someone that has not been working with your child complete this form, but we know that sometimes that is difficult to do. However, if that is possible, this person may be more objective than you might be. You will notice that this form has you rate the areas that we are most interested in, on a 7-point scale that is described in the form itself. The form is divided into global areas, and then further divided into specific communication areas so we can evaluate all of the features in which we are interested.

Clinical Global Impression Scale: Meta-play Version (Modified)

Child's Name:_____

Date:_____

INSTRUCTION: Please rate each of the 13 target symptom areas listed below, based on your impressions of the severity of your child's symptoms in these areas. Please use the "Impressions Rating Scale" listed below to make your daily ratings. At the end of the scheduled time period, circle your ratings below for each symptom area. It is important that each symptom area is rated. Try to use the same person (e.g., mother or father) to make the ratings.

Impression Rating Scale

1	= very much improved	4	= no change
2	= much improved	5	= minimally worse
3	= minimally improved	6	= much worse
		7	= very much worse

Global Symptom Areas

1.	Behavior Problems	1	2	3	4	5	6	7
2.	Responds to Social Interactions	1	2	3	4	5	6	7
3.	Initiates Social Interactions	1	2	3	4	5	6	7
4.	Use of Speech to Communicate	1	2	3	4	5	6	7
5.	Repetitive Behaviors	1	2	3	4	5	6	7
6.	Activity Level	1	2	3	4	5	6	7
7.	Nighttime Sleep	1	2	3	4	5	6	7

Specific Social Communication Areas

1.	Imitation (Doing what parent does)	1	2	3	4	5	6	7
2.	Gestures (Waving, shrugging etc.)	1	2	3	4	5	6	7
3.	Pointing (Pointing at objects or people)	1	2	3	4	5	6	7
4.	Showing (Showing objects spontaneously)	1	2	3	4	5	6	7
5.	Giving (Giving objects to another person)	1	2	3	4	5	6	7
6.	Responding to name (Responding when name is called)	1	2	3	4	5	6	7

Description of Each Target Symptom Area (for Global Symptoms):

1. *Behavior problems*: This item refers to occurrences of problem behaviors such as tantrums, aggression, property destruction, self-injury, mouthing, screaming, and running away.

2. ***Responds to social interactions***: This item refers to how well or how much your child responds to social interactions directed specifically to him or her.

3. ***Initiates social interactions***: This item refers to how well or how much your child independently uses initiates any type of social interactions.

4. ***Use of speech to communicate***: This item refers to how well or how much your child independently uses speech to communicate his/her wants, needs, desires, or feelings.

5. ***Repetitive behaviors***: This item refers to how well or how much your child spends engaged in repetitive behaviors such as: rocking, spinning, hand flapping, finger movements, covering/shielding eyes or ears, hoarding or arrangement of items, insisting on fixed routines or rituals, repetitive use of a specific toy or item, echolalia or repetitive sounds, words or phrases.

6. ***Activity level***: This item refers to the extent to which your child is overactive, hyperactive, "on the go"

7. ***Nighttime sleep***: This item refers to how much trouble your child has with sleeping through the night/getting a good night's sleep. Problems in this area could include difficulty going to sleep, frequently getting up during the night, or difficulty waking up in the morning.

Our research on the efficacy of the Meta-play Method is ongoing, and at some point in the future, I hope to say that this approach has been empirically shown to be effective. But this research will take many years to complete. In the meantime, I have compiled the activities of the Meta-play Method and the forms that we use in our research project in this manual for two reasons. First, it is a guide for parents who have chosen to engage in our research project. Second, I wanted to make these materials available for parents who choose to implement the Meta-play Method prior to the completion of our research, and any follow-up research that may take place. If the Meta-play Method does show some effectiveness, this second set of parents will have had a chance to help their children at a critical point in development. Our hope is that by basing our interventions on a theory that makes sense, we will be able to change the developmental trajectory of young children with autism so that the actual core symptoms are lessened or eliminated altogether. By intervening with focused strategies at the point in development theorized in DBTA to be critical to the ability to "think about," we hope to ignite the capacity to imagine and stop the cascading effects known as autism.

References

Dawson, G., Rogers, S., Munson, J., Smith, M., Winter, J. Greenson, J., Donaldson, A., & Varley, J. (2012). Randomized, controlled trial of an intervention for toddlers with autism: The Early Start Denver Model. Pediatrics, 125(1), e17-e23.

Dawson, G. (2012). Keynote lecture presented at Brown University, Lipsitt-Duchin Lecture Series on Child and Youth Behavior Development. May 1, 2012.

Hobson, P. (2002). The cradle of thought. New York: Oxford University Press.

Klin, A. Lin, D. L., Gorrindo, P., Ramsay, G., & Jones, W. (2009). Two-year-olds with autism orient to non-social contingencies rather than biological motion. *Nature, 459* (7244), 257-261.

National Institute of Mental Health. CGI Clinical Global Impression Scale – NIMH. *Psychopharmacology Bulletin, 21,* 839-844.

Sandler, A. D., Sutton, K. A., DeWeese, J. Giardi, M. A., Sheppard, V., & Bodfish, J. W. (1999). Lack of benefit of a single dose of synthetic human secretin in the treatment of autism and pervasive developmental disorder. *New England Journal of Medicine, 341 (24)*, 1801-1806.

CPSIA information can be obtained at www.ICGtesting.com
Printed in the USA
BVOW011522091112

305144BV00007B/18/P